Acclaim for
Tale of an Old Katfish

"John has been a tireless advocate for people with arthritis. He encourages all of us to support the fight for a better life for the more than 50 million Americans who live daily with the effects of arthritis. John's deeply personal perspective sheds light on the impact of the disease and on how a single individual can change the way others perceive it."

—Helen Emery, M.D., pediatric rheumatologist

———

"An inspiring account of one man's lifelong personal and public struggles with the health-care, judicial, and political bureaucracies through advocacy for his clients—adopted Katfish—as well as for himself."

—Jon Stevenson, M.D., rheumatologist

———

"This poignant memoir about how the love of family and friends sustains us in the face of adversity speaks to each reader in a special way. John's story will inspire and bring hope, not only to victims of juvenile arthritis but to all who suffer from a chronic medical condition."

—Maureen McGuire, Attorney at Law

———

"I have seen firsthand John's bravery and determination; he has dedicated his life to energizing our political leaders to help the millions who suffer. John's memoir is a story of how one man can stand against the odds and make a difference. It's an inspiration that will touch your heart."

—Congresswoman Cathy McMorris Rodgers,
5th District, Washington

———

"John Lynch's amazing journey and unwavering devotion are truly an inspiration. His tireless efforts have paved the way for all Katfish, and for this the Spokane JBR/W committee and all Katfish families will be forever grateful."

—Jeanne McCarty, Katfish mother

Tale of an Old Katfish

An Advocate's Memoir

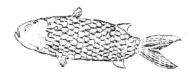

John P. Lynch

The
Rheumatoid Arthritis
Project

Tale of an Old Katfish
An Advocate's Memoir
Copyright © 2015 John P. Lynch

The Rheumatoid Arthritis Project
www.juvenilearthritisproject.org

Cover and book design by Cypress House
Front cover artwork by Christina McCarty
Author photo courtesy of Matt Lynch

Publisher's Cataloging-in-Publication Data

Lynch, John P. (John Patrick), 1947-

Tale of an old Katfish : an advocate's memoir / John P. Lynch. -- First edition. -- Spokane, WA : The Rheumatoid Arthritis Project, [2015]

pages ; cm.

ISBN: 978-0-9967077-0-1 (case) ; 978-0-9967077-1-8 (pbk)

Summary: At age eleven John Lynch was struck by juvenile rheumatoid arthritis, a crippling disease that affects 300,000 children. They are called Katfish, derived from Kids And Teens' Families Investing Support and Hope. Having found relief in a "miracle drug," John has dedicated his life to helping others who suffer from JRA. In addition to his journey from victim to advocate, this book tells the stories of young people fighting through pain and disability. Their stories will give hope and inspiration to anyone who must overcome seeming insurmountable obstacles to build successful lives.--Publisher.

1. Rheumatoid arthritis in children--Patients--Personal narratives. 2. Rheumatoid arthritis in children--Patients--Life skills guides. 3. Rheumatoid arthritis in children--Patients--Biography. 4. Rheumatoid arthritis--Patients--Personal narratives. 5. Rheumatoid arthritis--Patients--Life skills guides. 6. Chronically ill--Life skills guides. 7. Children with disabilities--Personal narratives. 8. Pain in children--Treatment. 9. Disability awareness. I. Rheumatoid Arthritis Project. II. Title.

RJ482.A77 L96 2015   2015951051

618.92/7227--dc23   1511

Printed in the USA
2 4 6 8 9 7 5 3 1
First edition

Disclaimer

I have tried to recreate events, locales, and conversations from my memories of them. In order to maintain their anonymity, I have in some instances changed the names of individuals and places, and may have changed some identifying characteristics and details such as physical traits, occupations, and places of residence.

Although the author and publisher have made every effort to ensure that the information in this book was correct at press time, the author and publisher do not assume and hereby disclaim any liability to any party for any loss, damage, or disruption caused by errors or omissions, whether such errors or omissions result from negligence, accident, or any other cause.

This book is not intended as a substitute for the medical advice of physicians. The reader should regularly consult a physician in matters relating to his/her health and particularly with respect to any symptoms that may require diagnosis or medical attention.

Dedicated to the cure for all Katfish,
and in appreciation of my family
and friends who helped me on my path.

Contents

Preface

What are Katfish? They are "Kids and Teens' Families Investing Support and Hope" for children with juvenile arthritis. Presently, there are 300,000 Katfish kids and teens in America afflicted by this painful, chronic, and disabling condition.

This is my tale of battling and, to some extent, overcoming juvenile arthritis. Many people have physical handicaps to overcome—birth defects, diseases, chronic conditions—that make life more difficult for them than for "normal" people. Living through the pain, the suffering, the shame, the frustration, and the sorrow of dealing with these "fallacies" is something I fully understand and attempt to chronicle my journey with juvenile arthritis in this advocate's memoir. My story is one of very many. I have put pen to paper in order to give inspiration to the many children, parents, and adults who daily battle their infirmities in an attempt to achieve their dreams.

As an old Katfish, my mission in telling this tale is to raise awareness about juvenile arthritis. By so doing I hope to continue helping in the search for the cure for juvenile arthritis, thereby making the Katfish like the dinosaur—a thing of the past! Until this happens, all Katfish must carry on as best they can. May the path I found for myself, through failure and success, show them one way it was done. If the reader takes away one thing from my memoir, please let it be "Don't give up—don't ever give up."

Chapter 1

Childhood – Before Juvenile Arthritis

Lawyers, I suppose, were children once.
—Charles Lamb

"It's a blond," the doctor dryly noted as I entered this world.

"John Patrick is his name!" exclaimed my mother at hearing the announcement.

"Just a minute, Mrs. Lynch," the doctor said. "We don't know yet if it's a boy."

In due course, however, the confusion was cleared up, but in the era before ultrasound, being named before being sexed must have been an unusual event in the delivery room. Regardless, my life outside the womb began as the second son of Jim and Margaret Lynch on July 9, 1947 in Spokane, Washington. Of the eleven years thereafter, the only remarkable feat I remember was playing in two tackle football games for St. Augustine's Parochial School on the same day.

These contests were accorded a single paragraph in our daily bugles, the *Spokesman-Review* and the *Spokane Daily Chronicle.* It was the first time—other than my birth announcement—that I, at least at a team level, received publicity. It would not be the last.

Until this noteworthy event took place, my first remembrance happened about the age of three. My brother, Jim, had two pet rabbits he kept caged. I suppose my independent bent manifested itself then because I thought they needed "extercize," whereupon I released them. This was a mistake for both the rabbits and me. One ran away, never to be seen again, and the other met its demise at the business end of a neighbor's dog. I'm sure I was disciplined, but the punishment I justly deserved then is beyond recall now. Such was my dear parents' gentle way of correcting my errant behavior.

Born between the bookends of my brother and my younger sister, Shannon, I expended a considerable amount of time, from her birth until high school, either trying to rid myself of this troublesome sibling, fending off my brother's less frequent but similar attempts upon me, or mixing it up with neighborhood kids and schoolyard foes. Such was my fate as a middle child, but these experiences, whether as victor or as vanquished, toughened me for the challenges ahead.

My sense of adventure led to spending a lot of time in the three public parks near my home: Comstock Park, Cannon Hill Park, and the crown jewel of all Spokane parks, Manito Park. Manito is the Algonquin native people's word that means the "deified spirit or force of nature," either good or bad. Spokane, named for the Spokan native people, means "children of the sun."

Manito Park and Spokane played a significant role in my life. By living in Spokane and playing in its sunny parks, I developed my body through swimming, skating, sledding, and football. I learned how to swim at Comstock because my mother insisted on it, and at Cannon Hill I taught myself how to ice skate and play hockey when its pond froze in the winter. It was Manito, however, the largest and prettiest of the three, where I spent a great deal of my youth. It was less than one block from home. Manito, Comstock, and Cannon Hill offered all of the space and freedom I needed to play, especially football. This challenging, but exciting game inevitably led to my first career choice: playing linebacker for the Baltimore Colts. Having started with the pads, cleats, and helmet in the autumn of fifth grade at Cannon Hill, I eagerly looked forward to the end of summer, even though it also meant the beginning of a new school term.

Chapter 2

Transition – Living with Arthritis

It was the best of times. It was the worst of times.
—Charles Dickens

In addition to getting better at football during the autumn of sixth grade, I actually liked a new school subject: history. As school was not my forte, it was a pleasant surprise to discover this classroom interest. It was innate, though, because my father had enjoyed it, too. My appreciation of the subject thus derives from the same genuine curiosity he had during his life of notable people and events from the past. So began a promising school year. I even took over my brother's *Spokane Daily Chronicle* paper route and made some money. Yes, life looked good indeed.

As the seasons changed from fall to winter and from winter to spring, I began to suffer physical pain from sore and swollen hands, knees, and feet. It was at its worst on awakening each day, but by the afternoon it temporarily subsided. I told no one because I didn't know better. I wanted to continue the school year the way it had started. Such, however, was not to be, for on a family vacation at an Idaho hot spring in May 1959, the cat leapt out of the bag. It was then that my mother, a registered nurse, discovered the telltale signs.

After arriving home the next port of call was the family doctor's office. His diagnosis was rheumatic fever, which at the time was a major concern of American parents. Dreaded like polio, it strikes children between the ages of five and fifteen. It is often evidenced by a sore throat brought on by an infection with streptococcus bacteria. Symptoms include fever, arthritis, and inflammation of the heart. Inflammation consists of redness, swelling, heat, and pain. The inflammatory process is the immune system's response when a foreign invader threatens the body. In some individuals this process leads to heart problems that require surgery. I didn't develop such problems, but even though my strep throat abated, the inflammatory symptoms, to one degree or another, continued.

The doctor's prescription was oral penicillin and bed rest. Little did I know at the time that the prognosis for full recovery was not possible. Being confined to bed, especially for the summer, felt like a life sentence, and with the all too frequent and painful blood draws by my physician, the winter of my discontent had unseasonably and irrevocably set in. As I grew older, there were many such winters, some lasting for years at a time.

During the summer of 1959, my hiatus from normal living evoked highs and lows I hadn't experienced before. My mother and my father's sister, Ramona, relieved the boredom by providing me with entertaining gifts. Rock and roll music had become popular, so I began listening to it on the radio. Mother picked up on this and, in addition to buying a record player, she let me get a new 45-rpm single every week. I would call the music department of the local Bon Marche for my selection, which would then be delivered. In addition to this delight, Aunt Ramona mailed weekly presents from Indiana, mostly model airplanes and ships, which I would eagerly assemble. These kindnesses of my mother and my aunt were good morale boosters.

Before reaching these peaks of contentment I went through the valleys of depression. I could no longer play outside with my friends, and except for my best buddy, Paul Tusch, no one visited me regularly. Maybe they didn't want to see me in pain. Maybe they were afraid my condition was contagious. Whatever the reasons, I was isolated from my classmates and neighborhood friends. The compulsory convalescence took a great toll, both physically and emotionally. As I reflect upon it now, however, it was the beginning of the development of my independence, a trait that would help me time and again.

It was also the beginning of a most meaningful and lifelong relationship neither Paul nor I could have foreseen. We were just a couple of pre-adolescent boys who lived the day. Paul understood my condition and what awaited me, but he didn't tell me because he wanted me to be upbeat. Although I couldn't play outside in the rough n' tumble way we were both used to, it didn't matter to Paul. We found other diversions, like listening to my records, playing chess, trading baseball cards, and talking the way sixth grade boys do; not yet about girls. That was a year or two away, but we were mischievous at times. We played some naughty tricks involving anonymous phone calls to numbers picked randomly from the directory. It was good-natured, and we got the poor listeners to participate unwittingly in our pranks. It was fun! As the reader will learn later, Paul became a wonderful advocate for the disabled. He had whatever effective advocate must possess: empathy.

Following my lengthy convalescence, the prescription remained the same: oral penicillin each day. I can't be certain how long I remained on this regimen, but it's likely it lasted until I left home for college. Also, I can't be certain whether the diagnosis of rheumatic fever was correct. In 1959 a diagnosis of juvenile arthritis was very difficult to make, and the treatments for it, if there had been any, were more limited than those for inflammatory arthritis in adults. Like Sherman's army plundering through the South on their relentless and devastating march to Savannah in 1864, the inflammation continued to wage unrelenting war on my joints.

Chapter 3

Adolescence

Neither fish nor fowl.
—Margaret Lynch, R.N.

Although others may claim the foregoing expression as their own, I attribute it to my mother. She was fond of using it to describe her adolescent offspring. It says what a teenager is—no longer a child but not yet an adult. In this respect my adolescence was no different, but my impaired body added a challenge I still refused to accept as part of my life.

As the new school year succeeded my convalescence, I actually looked forward to returning. I didn't start on the first day of the term, but entered seventh grade toward the end of September. Hoping to resume my former activities without a hitch, I once again turned out for football. During the prior season I had played quite well, especially on defense, so it was just a matter of honing my skills to a finer point. Was I wrong! Not only could I not play like I had, but I was cut from the team. Eyes bloodshot from tears, I walked slowly home and told my mother what had happened. My father wasn't there, so Mother had to console me by herself, but being one of nine offspring, a pediatric nurse, and a mother of four children (her first child, Betty Ann, having died in infancy), she responded with a mixture of love and toughness. Yes, it was terrible to be denied the chance to do what I really liked, but my young life would go on. It would be different, though—and so it was.

My intellectual curiosity having been teased to life by the subject of history, and my physical activities having been curtailed by my condition, I began to journey on another path. I suppose I had no choice. My parents provided me with the freedom to explore a different way of growing up. They did it, though, in a generally neutral way, neither encouraging nor discouraging most of my various forays. Whether by design, default, or both, they let me exercise my judgment and took over the helm only when a course correction required it. Like Darwin on shore leave during his revolutionary voyage aboard the *Beagle,* I was pretty much left to my own devices in the discovery of how to deal with my condition.

Upon reuniting with my classmates, I wanted to be treated the same way I had been before. At first it seemed possible. Despite the loss of playing organized sports, I maintained old friendships and cultivated new ones, but the physical limitations my malady imposed began to chip away at the healthy body I was born with. No longer one of the leaders of the pack, I slowly began my evolution into a lone wolf. I still enjoyed being with my friends and was even active in Boy Scouts, but the circle of my comrades slowly and inevitably tightened.

Not knowing what lay ahead of me insofar as my condition and treatment were concerned, but buoyed by the optimism of a twelve-year-old boy's spirit, I began to tackle other interests. My seventh grade teacher, a Franciscan nun, kept a fresh water aquarium in the classroom. I found the tropical fish so fascinating that I got a used tank and started my own school of guppies, zebra fish, black mollies, angelfish, tetras, catfish, and betas. I learned a lot from observing and taking care of them. The initial cost of acquiring my aquarium paled in comparison to maintaining it and replenishing my stock of fish, but taking care of them was further development of my responsibility to others, which had been seeded by my paper route.

As seventh grade flowed into eighth grade and the last year of parochial school into my first graduation, my impaired body added a challenge I still refused to accept, and for a long time thereafter. This forced change in my life's course, however, was producing a keener interest in academic pursuits. Thus when I entered high school in the fall of 1961, the honors program into which I had been enrolled became grist for my new mill. I still participated in extracurricular activities, such as debating on the freshman team, writing for the school newspaper, competing in elocution contests, attending Friday night football games, and being president of the school's service club, but outside of these activities and classes, I devoted each weekday evening to at least two hours of homework. I didn't know then why I suddenly liked studying. It may have been the honors setting or the challenge of new subjects such as Latin, chemistry, and classical Greek but I believe now that subconsciously it was my inability to play team sports. I had not given up physical activity. In fact Mother had encouraged me to learn snow skiing during the winter of 1960, which I continued until my late twenties. I even took up water skiing after my parents had purchased a motorboat, but except for these rather rigorous activities and the occasional pick up softball or touch football game at Manito, Cannon Hill, and Comstock, my athletic prowess continued to deteriorate. I had no measurable relief from the swelling and pain.

Occasionally, when my mother detected the blues my condition washed over me, she would cite the ancient adage: "I cried because I had no shoes. Then I met a man who had no feet." It is a reminder of the importance of perspective, which a chronically ill person must have. In her youth, Mother witnessed the suffering of uncles who had returned from the battlefields of World War I, forever maimed by gas, shock, or shell. I sometimes think that her exposure to their agony was one of the principal reasons she was able to become such a competent, caring, and compassionate registered nurse.

During her career, my mother specialized in the treatment of children. Her ability to help them was honed during her nursing duties at what was then called Shriners Hospital for Crippled Children. Patients ranged from infants to adolescents, all of whom had either orthopedic or burn problems, many of which required surgery. From straightening of spines to amputation of limbs to grafting of skin, the care of these children was lengthy and hard. Dealing with this daily demanded "tough love" from Mother, and she did not leave it at the hospital when she came home. It was a great gift for me to receive because it tempered me for the trials and tribulations that lay ahead. Despite the persistence of my symptoms, two important non-academic and non-athletic events in my young life happened: the companionship of my first dog, Patrick, and a keen interest in the opposite sex. Between the two I was kept very busy. Both were great fun. I knew the latter endeavor was bound to develop, and by my junior year I fell in love, for the very first time, with Pauline.

I had dated other girls, but only with Pauline had I felt the deep passion that first-time romance always brings. I hoped our love for each other would continue in college, but it was doomed. When we graduated from high school and went to different universities far away from one another, our relationship sadly but inevitably ended.

As for Patrick, it was a different story. He was my companion for the rest of his life. Having arrived at adolescence with only fish for pets, I longed for a puppy. The chance to have one presented itself because of my mother's bridge group. One of her partners, a bright but eccentric lady, was very fond of Irish Setters. Shamrock, her prized possession, had been bred with a champion Irish Setter and then had a litter of several furry red pups. Mother was opposed to letting me have one, but between her bridge partner's acquiescence and my persistence, she relented. The runt of the litter became mine and we spent many days together, especially in Manito. Patrick was a joy to watch, running swiftly and gracefully, and it was sheer delight to play hide and seek, I as the hare and he the hound. For nine years he was an integral part of my life. I was lucky to have had him.

Chapter 4

College and Early Work Life

Things are seldom what they seem; skim milk masquerades as cream.
—William Gilbert and Arthur Sullivan

The classic couplet, memorialized in *HMS Pinafore,* was a harbinger of my young adulthood. Having shed adolescence like a snake its skin, my youthful optimism would be tempered by realism in the crucible of my post-secondary education and first full-time employment.

By graduating tenth in my high school class of 174, I earnestly believed that such academic success would continue at the collegiate level. Since professional football was out the question, medicine was my second career choice. With the nearest medical school at the University of Washington, I enrolled in their undergraduate chemistry program in the fall of 1965. My best friend, Paul, chose the UW too. We were the only seniors from Gonzaga Preparatory School to do so, despite the dire warning of our sociology teacher that it was "a pagan temple filled with godless communists." As it turned out, a much bigger problem lay in store for us: being far from home amid fierce competition.

Having been a big fish in a small pond, it was culture shock to have my ecosystem change so dramatically. Entry-level survey courses could be twice as large as my graduating class. Added to this terror was the relentless application of Darwin's theory of natural selection. With more than 20,000 undergraduates, it was every student for himself, and as if the scramble for earning good grades wasn't enough, there was the independence of dorm life impeding my progress. With no parental oversight, I didn't apply myself as I should have. By the end of my freshman year, I had barely managed to stay off academic probation. With such lack of scholastic achievement, I had virtually eliminated myself from ever being considered for medical school.

Granted, the curriculum my academic advisor had scheduled for me was daunting, but a career as a physician is no less so, and even if I hadn't had the added difficulty of moving my impaired body across a large campus, it's doubtful I could have measured up to the rigorous requirements, both physical and intellectual, the medical profession demands. Although my grades improved as I adjusted to the competition and the independence, my untreated condition did not. One benefit, however, that the UW offered, which my hometown had not, was a large medical complex with specialists in rheumatic diseases. Consequently, during my sophomore year, the student health department referred me to the UW rheumatology department. Their diagnosis was juvenile rheumatoid arthritis and their prescription was twelve plain aspirin a day.

Juvenile rheumatoid arthritis (JRA), now known as juvenile idio-pathic arthritis (JIA), is a chronic, inflammatory autoimmune disease in which the body's immune system attacks the joints and other parts of the body, thereby causing chronic pain, suffering, and, if not diagnosed early and treated properly, permanent deformity. It is the most common type of arthritis that afflicts children and there are many forms of this dread disease. Mine is polyarticular because it has affected five or more joints on both sides of my body.

Aspirin has been used as a medicine since ancient times. Long ago, people discovered that eating willow tree bark or brewing a tea from it could be helpful for some illnesses. In the late 19th century, the active chemical in willow bark, salicylate, was synthesized as a pill. For temporary relief of pain and inflammation, aspirin remains today an effective drug, but plain aspirin is too irritating to the stomach for long-term use in the high quantities needed to treat JRA.

With it being the late 1960s and with my approaching adulthood, a prescription of aspirin for my JRA was probably appropriate. While I didn't have stomach irritation from taking such a large dosage of daily aspirin, ringing developed in my ears, but beyond aspirin there was nothing else that the UW medical specialists could do for me. Just like the rest of my life as a collegian, I was on my own on how to deal with my JRA.

Unknown to me at the time of my new diagnosis, the slow erosion of my joints continued unabated, particularly in my hands and feet, but the inflammatory process had lessened, so I learned to live with the morning stiffness and discomfort. The heavy dose of aspirin alleviated these symptoms, but its side effects eventually forced me from this therapy. Deviating temporarily from this and any other treatment, and undergoing certain radical medical regimens later on, would have profound and irreversible effects for the rest of my life.

Even though my relationship with Pauline had ended, my keen interest in women had not. I continued pursuing "the female of the species" with a young man's ardor. Relationships of varying duration and intensity came and went as I progressed toward a bachelor's degree in chemistry. By senior year I was getting ready to apply to medical school, but even with a solid science curriculum and a good GPA, my instincts told me the chances of acceptance were slim.

The same could not be said of my prospects for a long and meaningful relationship with Vivian. She is the daughter of the late Sol and Erika Levy. Just as my ancestors had fled the Irish potato famines of the 1840s, Vivian's parents had escaped the European fascism of the 1930s. They started life anew on America's East Coast and eventually settled in Spokane. From the tragedy of losing their parents in the Holocaust, they determined to do whatever it took to make the lives of their children safe and secure. Thus Vivian and her brother, Steve, grew up nurtured by the love of their parents who provided the best they could for their progeny. Theirs was a safe and comfortable childhood.

It was during my senior year that I met Vivian. She had recently transferred from the University of the Pacific to the UW, and we were returning there following our holiday break in Spokane. As we traveled by plane, which for me then was a very rare occasion, a mutual acquaintance introduced us. To our pleasant surprise, we discovered we were campus neighbors. This being so it was easy to see one another as often as we wanted. Our cadre of friends proved mutually accepting of Vivian and me, and we had lots of good times with them, especially my UW Rho Beta cluster brothers, Steve Bruno, affectionately known as Seb, Harold Rathman, Jack Lee, Tom Norman, Tommy Fong, and my roomie and good friend, the late Mike Tumlinson, affectionately known as MT. Nurtured by their companionship, the seeds of love blossomed for Vivian and me in the spring of 1969, but Vivian's being a sophomore and my graduating in June eventually led to our separation. Unlike the aftermath of my high school graduation, however, our relationship would not only survive being apart, but would also thrive with the passage of time. Four more years, however, would pass before our reunification.

Despite improving my grades and adapting more responsibly to undergraduate life, I knew that admission to medical school was unlikely. Nonetheless, I applied to a dozen or so throughout the country. When the last of the rejections arrived, however, I was faced with going to work as a chemist or trying my hand in a new field. I opted for the latter and ended up in the MBA program at the University of Oregon. Since I had had no business school courses, I was required to take core undergraduate classes in marketing, finance, personnel management, economics, computer science, and accounting. The last of these proved to be the field I would enter upon graduation. Before I enrolled in the MBA program, I had to deal with another major milestone in my life. On turning eighteen in the summer of 1965, I registered with the U.S. Selective Service System. Mandated for all men by federal law, even teenagers eighteen and older, this registration was the primary source for conscription—better known as the draft—into the American armed forces. Ultimately, American college students and others opposed to the Vietnam War succeeded in bringing about enactment of the 26th Amendment to the U.S. Constitution, which lowered the voting age from twenty-one to eighteen. Teenagers can still be conscripted, but they can now vote for their congressional representatives who determine whether America can declare war. Now Congress is more circumspect about using this ultimate power of the federal government to put men and women of the armed forces "in harm's way."

At the time I registered, I didn't have a say in whether I could be drafted because I couldn't vote until I turned twenty-one. With the country's military involvement in Vietnam steadily increasing, a lottery system based on birth dates determined the fate of men and teenagers—the lower one's number, the greater the chance of being shipped off to Vietnam courtesy of the U.S. Army—for at least two years. It didn't mean much to me then because in the fall of 1965, I had begun my college education. This pursuit automatically deferred my eligibility for the draft.

Upon completing my undergraduate studies in 1969, that deferment expired, but the war in Vietnam was raging then, and because of America's commitment, casualties were mounting significantly. Thus there was even more pressure from the armed forces to fill their depleted ranks through the draft. In light of this the Selective Service System summoned me for a medical examination. If found fit for duty, I was subject to induction into the army with a better than even chance of going to Vietnam.

At the time of my examination I informed the Selective Service physician of my arthritis, but the abnormalities it had caused were not obvious. My finger joints were somewhat enlarged, but their deterioration was not marked. I could still use them, but along with my wrists, knees, ankles, and feet there was chronic pain and impairment of function. Even with these signs and symptoms, the examining physician apparently discounted my limitations. Whether it was because I was young and, in his opinion, not likely to have arthritis or because of some other reason not disclosed to me, it was *pes planus* (flat feet) that kept me from being drafted. Ironically, they were caused by the lack of physical activity during my five-month bed confinement in 1959. I mention this episode because in 1969, and for a considerable time thereafter, many people, doctors included, believed arthritis was an old-age affliction. Infants, children, adolescents, and even young adults did not get this disease. I don't know why the draft-board physician found flat feet, rather than arthritis, the basis for my disqualification. I suppose there weren't many young people like me then. I certainly didn't know anyone in my generation who had arthritis, but JRA was the real reason why I wasn't conscripted.

Unlike some of my high school classmates who were found fit and shipped off to Vietnam, JRA kept me out of its rice paddies and jungles. While I didn't have to confront the threat of violent injury or death on its battlefields, I sometimes ponder why I was spared that fate on the far side of the world.

The two years spent in graduate school were less stressful and more satisfying than the previous four as an undergraduate. Further, except for a brief stint in the dorm, I experienced apartment life for the very first time. This meant learning how to buy groceries, cook from scratch, and keep the bathroom relatively hygienic. I also discovered the beautiful Oregon Coast. While I was not dealing with my JRA like I should have, my mental outlook improved a lot, but what helped most was seeing Vivian as frequently as I could, despite having no car and her living 250 miles away. This inevitably meant taking the Greyhound red-eye on Friday evening and arriving at the UW campus shortly after midnight.

As my second-quarter final exams were about to conclude, I chanced upon an opportunity that would have significant consequences. Professor Dale Harwood, one of my accounting professors, gave the class the choice of either taking the standard test or writing a paper. I opted for the latter. That effort improved my grade, and according to his letter accompanying my paper, Professor Harwood said it was "the only one worth its salt." He then went on to ask where and why I'd been hiding myself under a bushel basket. At the close of his letter, he wrote, "Have been trying to recall your undergrad major. Was it chemistry? If it was and you can write the way you do, you've got it made, whatever direction you take."

I had never had any teacher ask me so important a question. Per Professor Harwood's suggestion, I did an independent research paper for him and interviewed with the U.S. General Accounting Office. Upon graduating with my MBA degree in the spring of 1971, I accepted a position with this congressional auditing agency, but my place of employment would be San Francisco, thus putting me even farther away from Vivian.

I spent three years in San Francisco performing field audits of federal programs, both military and civilian, for the GAO. Sometimes temporary duty stations meant giving up my apartment for quarters in far-flung places such as Reno, Nevada, and Portland, Oregon. My tour of duty in Portland provided the necessary experience for obtaining a CPA license and the opportunity to be with Vivian in Spokane on many a weekend. Though I thought that accounting would be the source of my life's earnings, I found the bureaucracy and office politics too hard to handle. Before I decided to leave, I proposed to Vivian and she accepted.

We were married by Rabbi Eli Burkow, the San Francisco State University Jewish chaplain, and Father LeRoy Weeks, the St. Augustine Church assistant Catholic priest, on May 27, 1973. I believe that the ceremony, celebrated before a large gathering of family and friends, both Christian and Jewish, in the Ridpath Hotel, was the first of its kind in Spokane. Our wedding was a very memorable occasion and lots of fun, and just after we broke the glass beneath the canopy, Rabbi Burkow declared to all of our guests, "You don't have to be Jewish to say, 'Mazel tov!'"

Chapter 5

Law School

The mills of the gods are late to grind, but they grind small.
—Sextus Empiricus

Little did I realize or appreciate what being married really meant until my first day in the mill of law school. Even our four-year courtship leading up to matrimony did not properly prepare Vivian and me for the life of a married couple. Our first year alone in San Francisco, far from family and friends, was nevertheless fairly stress free. Both of us were gainfully employed in our fields, she as a social worker and I as a supervisory auditor. We cultivated new relationships with coworkers and enjoyed occasional explorations of the Bay Area.

The growing dissatisfaction with my work gnawed at me to such an extent that I decided to take the law school admission test. Upon receiving the results, I applied to several law schools. The most promising prospect was Gonzaga University School of Law in our hometown. Following a personal interview with one of the professors on the admissions committee, I was accepted for enrollment. After three years of government service, I entered law school in the fall semester of 1974.

Being twenty-seven years old and having had a certain amount of real-life experience, I was not one of the typical first-year day-school students. Most of them were single and fresh out of college with a bachelor's degree. My being married barely a year and having been out of school more than three seemed to outweigh, at least in the beginning, the advantages of age, a master's degree, and prior employment.

Regardless, in law school I learned the curriculum through the time-tested Socratic method. Still used in legal classrooms today, this method is named for the philosopher Socrates. He taught students by asking question after question, seeking to expose contradictions in the thoughts and ideas of his charges. By so doing, his goal was to guide them to a logical conclusion.

More often than not, my law school professors selected their targets at random for this rigorous classroom exercise. To be as prepared as much as possible, I spent long, arduous hours briefing cases assigned by my professors, analyzing the facts and law for the topic *du jour* for the next class, and then debating these learned men and women when picked out to stand on my hind legs for the inevitable milling. The classic film, *The Paper Chase*, which graphically underscores my point, should be required viewing for anyone who's even thinking about law school. If you are admitted to the halls of legal academe, never let it be said that you weren't forewarned—and trust me: By the end of your first year you will turn into a cynical masochist, unless you were one already. Fear not, however, those students fated to transition from the darkness to the light! Patience must be your mantra. You still must graduate, pass the onerous bar exam, pay off your outrageous law school loans, and survive the lean years of your law practice. If you do all of these and finally reap the rewards of becoming a member of the bar, you will leave this earthly coil free from the shackles of the Frankenstein Monster, Cynical Masochist.

With virtually all of my waking time devoted to the mind-numbing monotony of briefing endless cases, my relationship with Vivian began to deteriorate. Fortunately, we had no children then, but the strain of my studies was hurting both of us. The first-year courses were, with the exception of torts, boring. As a result, non-academic endeavors came to a virtual standstill. Life indeed had become drudgery. By the end of that year, I understood all too well the skepticism Sextus Empiricus, another philosopher, had espoused in his treatise "Against the Professors," but then a break in the mills of my professors ensued. I entered the eye of the law school hurricane.

My father-in-law learned that Judge William H. Williams, a well-known and well-respected member of the Spokane County Superior Court bench, needed a fill-in bailiff for the summer. After a year's hiatus, I reentered the work force and found the courtroom experience valuable on-the-job training. In addition to handling Judge Williams's docket, I dealt with other judges, their staff, attorneys, juries, parties, witnesses, and the press. After my predecessor passed the bar exam, the position opened for year-round employment. I therefore continued as a daytime bailiff during the remainder of my law school experience and evolved into a creature of the night. Once again the dial of chance spun favorably, at least as far as my marriage was concerned—but not so for my health.

I was now twenty-eight, and had been afflicted with JRA for a full seventeen years. Though still young, my untreated condition was producing subtle and destructive changes, and while I had begun seeing a specialist in rheumatic diseases, his course of treatment proved too costly. To begin with, he prescribed drugs that were far stronger than aspirin. In point of fact, their toxic side effects worsened my condition. His approach to my disease accorded with the general change in the treatment of rheumatoid arthritis: from conservative to aggressive; but my failure to respond to each and every one of his poisonous potions significantly increased the unwarranted risk not only of my permanent disability, but also more important, my premature death.

I was beginning to feel like a foot soldier in "Unconditional Surrender" Grant's campaign of 1865. Like the hard-drinking, cigar-smoking general relentlessly pursuing Bobby Lee throughout Virginia, my rheumatologist threw at me every available weapon to win the war against my JRA, and just like Grant's foot soldiers who miraculously survived his bloody strategy but were permanently scarred by near death and needless suffering, so did I. The culmination of the disastrous rheumatologist's treatment was his recommendation that I undergo a synovectomy of the large knuckles of my left hand. This surgical procedure removes the synovial tissue that encapsulates the joint. Inside this lining is the synovial fluid, which, like oil for an engine, lubricates the joint for easy movement.

I had tried operations twice before. Taking out tonsils and adenoids had once been advocated as a way to treat JRA. I don't know why, but Mother, a very experienced RN, permitted it, and so as a teenager I underwent what was then considered routine surgery for youngsters–whether they had JRA or some other condition for which this invasive procedure was routinely prescribed. It did me no good. Later, while living in San Francisco, I underwent a bunionectomy of my right big toe. Unlike my tonsils and adenoids, the bunion has since grown back. Regardless, the synovectomy not only failed to alleviate my JRA but also caused permanent impairment and deformity in my left hand. This medical mistake would have other far-reaching consequences. The only good outcome from my rheumatologist's medical malpractice was ridding myself of him forever. I then came under the care of a conservative, older internist, the late Robert Johnson, M.D., a kind, caring, and compassionate physician who put me on a weaker drug regimen. It helped because it was really the only option then. The legacy of this good doctor lives on in his sons, also kind, caring, and compassionate physicians, Mark Johnson, M.D., my primary care physician, and his brother, Stephen Johnson, M.D., an internist as well. Both are genuine doctors in the best traditions of the medical profession.

When I finished law school, my next step before admission to the legal profession was sitting for the bar examination. I was thirty years old and this lengthy test proved to be more of a challenge than just my knowledge about the law. The progression of arthritis had caused more joint erosion and pain, particularly in my hands and wrists. I had already undergone surgery on my left hand during my second year in law school, so I knew I would be at a physical disadvantage in writing my answers. With two and a half days devoted to the exam, something had to be done to deal with my limitation.

As it turned out, a local attorney and friend of my parents advised them that I could take the exam by dictating my answers. I followed his advice and contacted the Washington State Bar Association. They required a medical certificate attesting to the physical impairment in my hands and wrists. My physician provided a certificate in which he stated that JRA put me at a physical disadvantage with respect to the other examinees. Consequently, arrangements were made for me to dictate my answers, which were then transcribed. I reviewed the transcription for any errors or supplementation, made the necessary revisions, and then submitted my answers. Three months after finishing the bar exam, the Washington State Supreme Court admitted me to practice as an attorney at law.

The reason I mention this experience is because it is one way I learned to level the uneven field of endeavor. I took advantage of an opportunity because my life had been adversely affected by JRA. It was hard enough dealing daily with the physical pain and mental anguish this chronic condition causes and then confronting the challenges any professional career presents. Without the aid of dictation and transcription, I mighty very well have failed the bar exam; but with the help of my parents' friend, my physician, and the bar association, I passed. From this episode in my life with JRA, I urge all Katfish to take advantage of every opportunity that can put them on equal footing with the able-bodied.

Chapter 6

Lawyer and Father

The ever-whirling world of change.
—Edmund Spenser

In the spring of 1978, Vivian and I bought our first home. It was a starter house in the Downriver area of Spokane. About seven miles from our parents' homes, this lovely neighborhood was where we began our family. We had heard of Downriver, but knew little about it. It wasn't long before we came up to speed and discovered one of its treasures: It's a great incubator and nursery. Other young neighborhood couples found this out too. Before long, babies were popping out everywhere. It was like a rabbit warren.

Shortly after leaving the home of Vivian's parents where we spent most of our time during the law school years, two momentous but inevitable changes occurred in the life cycle of our family: the death of Vivian's father and the birth of our first child, Monica.

Upon return from a trip to the Galapagos Islands, Sol, who had just turned sixty-eight, was diagnosed with multiple myeloma, an agonizing and lethal form of cancer. While Vivian and I did not realize then it was a death sentence, we are now certain that Sol did. Nonetheless, he underwent grueling and painful treatment, and continued treating his patients nearly to the end of his life. Despite the dread prognosis, he also learned Vivian was pregnant with Monica. It was his expressed wish that he live to see the birth of his second grandchild. Sadly, it went unfulfilled, and he died on October 31, 1978. Monica was born three months later.

Before these seminal events, I had begun to establish my practice as a private attorney, essentially on my own. I did share expenses, such as rent, secretary, and telephone, with my two colleagues, Larry Butler and Mark Conlin. With the exception of mutual clients, however, we didn't split fees, and lacking clientele out of the gate, my income was for the first year, to put it charitably, very modest.

What a young lawyer lacks in experience and lots of paying clients he can usually overcome with optimism, a willingness to take on any case, and just plain good luck. I had all three going for me. Besides, what else could I do? The die had been cast and it was now sink or swim. Being a naturally good swimmer, I kept my head above water, and, like Julius Caesar had done many centuries ago, I pulled for the far shore of my own Rubicon and did not turn back. I had no other choice.

Just after I announced to family, friends, and anyone else who would listen that I was available for legal consultation and engagement, Judge Williams asked me to be his campaign treasurer. Having served nearly twenty years as superior court judge, he had decided to run for the elective position of justice of the state supreme court. A natural politician with credentials as a boxer, college quarterback, bomber pilot, and deputy prosecuting attorney, he stood a strong chance of getting his bottom on the state court's top bench, but he needed someone to manage his war chest. With an MBA degree and a CPA license, I was the most likely candidate to fill the unpaid position of money manager. Since I couldn't say no, I signed on.

If it had been a simple matter of accounting for Judge Williams's campaign contributions and expenses, I'd have had a lot less stress in carrying out this extracurricular activity, but such was not the case. In the mid-1970s, Congress and the state legislatures reacted to the Watergate fiasco and the resignation of President Richard Nixon with stringent campaign finance reform laws. As a result public disclosure commissions were created, which in turn adopted reporting requirements that generated mountains of deadline-driven paperwork.

Although ignorance can be bliss, the last thing Judge Williams needed was any kind of snafu for his campaign finance reporting. This meant my initial unfamiliarity with filing timely and accurate reports of what he received and how he spent it, especially in a non-partisan, three-way judicial race, would simply not do. Therefore I had to come up to speed quickly and make sure that at least my part in the campaign complied with the state laws and the rules of the newly minted Public Disclosure Commission. I did not let the judge down.

Being an east-sider in a state where 80 percent of the population lives on the west side posed a particularly difficult challenge for Judge Williams, but his two primary opponents hailed from the other side of the Cascade Curtain, thus enabling him to divide and conquer. While judicial ethics prevent mudslinging during an election campaign, there's no prohibition against electioneering. The judge's campaign strategist, a former law partner and president of the Washington State Bar Association, was an experienced hand at politics, and with enough money raised for the race, the judge parlayed his personality, experience, and esteem into not only a primary triumph but also the ultimate prize itself in the general election. It was a bittersweet victory, though, for Vivian's mother: Being a close friend of the judge and his family, Erika was present with Vivian and me in the judge's home when the general election returns awarded him the position of associate justice, but the judge's victory had come right on the heels of Sol's funeral. Widowhood was now permanently part of her life, and she would live alone for the next twenty-five years. There was, however, the great expectation of another grandchild and once born, Monica filled the void immeasurably for her maternal grandmother. The bond Erika developed with our daughter was very special to both of them. Pure kismet!

After Vivian and I were married, but before Monica was conceived, we rarely discussed the issue of offspring. Her work and my legal education precluded any serious consideration of parenthood, but as our fourth anniversary approached, I had reached the milestone of completing law school. There were still other matters to which efforts would be directed: Studying for and taking the bar exam, touring Western Europe thereafter, and launching my career upon passing the bar, but what really led to the conception of our daughter was having our own home.

Thus on January 25, 1979, having been induced with drugs and pried loose with forceps, Monica was born early. Unlike my entry into the world, however, there was no doubt about her sex, but Vivian's prolonged labor and our daughter's prematurity took their toll: She had to spend time in an oxygen tent under the bilirubin light. Although she recovered from the jaundice, I believe the oxygen therapy adversely affected her vision. Regardless, I took Vivian and Monica home three days after delivery. She weighed less than five pounds. So began my life as a father.

Two years later our son, Matt, was born on January 3, 1981. His arrival took less than one hour from the time we left home until he was born. Vivian never got out of the labor room, and her ob-gyn arrived only after the delivery. Just as Matt made his way into this world, the nurse handed me the scissors and asked me if I wanted to cut his umbilical cord. I didn't hesitate. One clean snip and he was free from his mother. Our family was now complete.

With the opening of my practice and the arrival of our children, my stress level began to rise dramatically. Not only was there the pressure of keeping the doors of my office open but also I was now solely responsible for producing the family income. Following Monica's birth, Vivian stayed home until Matt was in the fourth grade. This meant ten years without her salary, but once we felt comfortable with our circumstances, Vivian resumed her profession. All of our family was very fortunate that she was able to stay home during this important time in our children's development.

Chapter 7

The Pressures of Life

None knows the weight of another's burden.
—George Herbert

Now into my third decade of living with arthritis, I began to deal with it more aggressively. Through a combination of pharmaceutical drugs and more surgery, I was hopeful I could at least stabilize my condition. With a new private practice and the onset of parenthood, there was no other option.

Little did I know what a roller coaster ride I would be on for the next eleven years. The hallmark of JRA is that it typically waxes and wanes between flares and remissions. Like a smoldering fire, it lies dormant. Many factors account for this, but the sad fact of the matter is it can't be extinguished, it can only be controlled, and when it erupts, as it inevitably does, its effects can be devastating.

In addition to the regimen of drugs and surgery, I used hydrotherapy, especially swimming, to deal with the daily stiffness and pain in my wrists, hands, ankles, and feet. I employed other treatment modalities such as daily whirlpool baths, dog walking, bicycling, and fixed-weight lifting. I even tried acupuncture, elimination of suspected inflammatory foods from my diet, and allergy shots. Mother injected me every week for what seemed an eternity. The shots stung like angry yellow jackets. Moreover, I reduced my weight and improved my limited range of motion. There was very little pain from JRA, and my medical treatment consisted of a single anti-inflammatory prescription drug. I was feeling so well that I began training for the swimming leg of the third annual Lake Coeur d'Alene Triathlon. Aptly named "The Scenic Challenge," which it truly is, the triathlon courses through the lake's warm waters, beside its beautiful shores, and high into the verdantly forested hills nearby. Participation in it with my brother and my nephew, Brian, signaled a major milestone in my life. I firmly believed I had finally fought the final battle with my nemesis to a stalemate. I had turned the corner and was headed in the right direction. The year was 1985.

With improvement in my health, I became more involved with my children. They had started their primary education at a nearby public school. Vivian and I supported their activities, both school-related and extracurricular, and with the arrival of youth soccer in America, I became one of their coaches. I also volunteered with the school's parent-teacher group, eventually serving as president. Other community activities included a term as board chairman of the local branch of the Children's Home Society of Washington and as one of the organizers of the Pittsburg Neighborhood Association. The association's sole purpose was the reclassification of South Pittsburg Street, where we raised our children, from designation as an arterial in the Spokane Arterial Street Plan to a local-access street. Reclassifying our street comported with the reality of the neighborhood's character and charm. Armed with the expertise of a good traffic engineer and a land-use lawyer, paid for by the generous contributions of South Pittsburg residents and the residents of the neighboring streets and avenues adversely affected by "The Plan," the association convinced the Spokane City Council to do "the politically correct thing." Thus the South Pittsburg Street neighborhood remains to this day "a nice place to live."

Coupled with the increased activity level in our family and community was the burgeoning of my law practice. Clients brought in complex litigation, both factual and legal. I therefore spent considerably more time battling "my worthy opponents." Representation of clients in court, especially those suffering serious injuries inflicted upon them by tortfeasors, was a key factor in this progression of my practice. In particular, one client's case almost took over my life. Resolution came only after seven hard years.

Chapter 8

The Odyssey of Gerald
and Virginia Wilson

Tell me, O Muse, of that ingenious hero who traveled far and wide after he had sacked the famous city of Troy. Many places did he visit, and many were the nations with whose manners and customs he was acquainted. Moreover, he suffered much while at sea trying to save his own life and bring his men home safely.

But do what he might he could not save his men, for they perished through their own sheer folly by eating the cattle of the Sun-god, Hyperion. So the god prevented them from reaching home.
Tell me, too, about all these things, Athena, O Daughter of Zeus, from what-soever source you may know them.

—Homer

My client, Gerald Wilson, true salt of the earth if ever there was one, and whom I had the distinct honor and privilege of representing in previous engagements, started on his own odyssey in 1984. Like the heroic Odysseus, he suffered much while trying to save his own life. Unlike Odysseus, who ultimately survived his twenty-year odyssey, Gerald, after a six-year ordeal, died from AIDS. The healthcare and justice systems had failed him.

In 1984 Gerald underwent the first of two elective knee-replacement surgeries. He had recently retired from a life of hard manual labor, and both of his arthritic knees were burned out because of it. I knew from first-hand experience what his working life had been like. When I was living at my parents' home, they paid Gerald to apply stain to the shingles on their roof. Going up and down the ladder was hard for him, especially to get a fresh bucket of stain, so I was assigned the task of preparing the stain on the ground and attaching the filled bucket to a rope. My parents didn't pay me for my hard labor. It was involuntary servitude, my room and board more than enough compensation for their undeserving son. Anyway, Gerald would then pull the bucket to the roof, thereby considerably reducing the number of times he had to climb up and down the ladder.

Following Gerald's surgery, a blood transfusion was ordered. The blood was contaminated with human immunodeficiency virus (HIV), the precursor to acquired immunodeficiency syndrome (AIDS). The sad irony of this tragic event is that Gerald had been a longtime donor to the local blood bank (now defunct), which had supplied the infected unit. In point of fact, during his lengthy history of donation, stretching back to the 1930s, he had donated more than ten gallons of blood. Had he known he could have had his own blood drawn and stored for his elective surgery, through the simple and safe process called autologous blood donation, he would have done so, but no one told him about this simple procedure.

From the records the blood bank was compelled to produce during the discovery phase of the litigation, I learned that their board of directors had discussed the risk of contamination of blood by the AIDS virus more than a year before Gerald's first surgery. In light of this risk, the board then recommended that local physicians be reminded of the blood bank's autologous blood policy. According to their own records, the blood bank did nothing further in this regard. Since Gerald's surgeon did not discuss the risk of transfusion-associated AIDS and the blood bank's autologous blood policy with him, he never had the chance to insure against the risk of infection through self-donation.

Nevertheless, Gerald underwent the knee operation. Apparently, it was uneventful and he tolerated the procedure well. Even though he lost about 500 cc of blood during the surgery, none was given to him at that time. Later the same day, the hospital notified the surgeon that Gerald's blood pressure had dropped significantly. The surgeon then ordered that Gerald be given two units of packed cells, one of which, as was later discovered, was infected with the AIDS virus. As a result of yet another "failure to communicate" vital information, the blood was transfused after Gerald's blood pressure had begun to rise. The transfusion was therefore unnecessary.

The AIDS epidemic was in its infancy when Gerald was infected with the tainted blood; so was the law in developing legal theories of recovery for transfusion-associated AIDS cases. With no effective treatment for this lethal disease at that time, Gerald was a dead man walking. He and his wife, Virginia, had been grievously injured and they wanted me to initiate a claim for damages. It would take more than six years to finally settle. Before the resolution of his case through mediation, Gerald bled to death from AIDS. The records of the "not for profit" blood bank revealed that once they found out just how badly they had blundered, they devised and implemented a brutal strategy against their loyal longtime donor.

For Katfish this is a significant story because it really started with arthritis. If Gerald had not developed such painful and crippling osteoarthritis in both knees, he would never have been operated on, and had he not been operated on, he would never have been infected with a deadly disease, but arthritis in this country has been constantly cast as "just part of getting old, so get used to it." No matter what form arthritis takes, it is a major health problem for all Americans afflicted with it.

When I was a child, children didn't get arthritis. Or so it seemed. It was as untrue then as it is now. Katfish must change this misperception because they have "skin in the game," that is, they have a vital stake in raising awareness about juvenile arthritis and finding the cure. Had Gerald's generation had the awareness of how awful arthritis can be, no matter how young or how old a person is, then maybe he would not have suffered needlessly and horribly. As the reader will learn later, Katfish are now making a significant difference, not only for themselves but also for millions of Americans—of all ages—because the chickens have come home to roost!

Chapter 9

The Failure of the Healthcare System

Let all the poisons that lurk in the mud hatch out!
—Claudius

When Claudius, the fourth Roman emperor, uttered this damning declaration, he was writing the history of his family. During his long life, purely because he played the family fool, Claudius survived the basest and most predatory behavior human beings are capable of. While the healthcare and justice systems did not intentionally kill Gerald, they did, beyond a shadow of a doubt, fail him. His odyssey proves why.

During his lifetime, Gerald donated ten gallons of blood to the blood bank. His history of donations began early in his life. His motivation for giving blood was simply because people needed it. In most instances, he never knew the recipients. On one occasion when he was a young man, he heard a radio request for his type of blood. Unable to afford the streetcar fare, he walked over a mile to the hospital. Upon arriving there, he was informed that they were not ready for him so he walked home. Later that day, he again walked to the hospital, gave his blood, and returned home the same way.

In addition to becoming a member of the Ten-Gallon Donor Club at the blood bank, Gerald gave at least twenty additional units in other places, thus bringing his lifetime level to over one hundred units of blood. This model behavior encouraged others to become donors. Further, as the chairman of his local union blood-bank committee, he arranged countless blood drives for the blood bank, which honored him with a public announcement and the display of his name on their Ten-Gallon Donor "Milk Can."

According to the blood bank's records, Gerald tested positive for the AIDS virus after his first surgery. Follow-up tests by the blood bank confirmed this diagnosis. The reason Gerald's blood had been tested was because he had resumed his normal routine of donating blood. Following the first post-surgery donation, he gave five more units, all of which tested positive for the AIDS virus. Despite these test results, which covered a ten-month period, no one from the blood bank informed him about them until nearly a year after the blood bank had first discovered his positive reaction to the virus!

The blood bank was just as callous to the donor, a young husband and father, about notifying him of his contaminated donation. In December 1985 the blood bank determined the donor's blood had been transfused into Gerald. The blood bank then called the donor on the pretext that his type of blood was needed. At the time of his donation, the blood bank did not tell him that his blood was being drawn just to test it. The surrogate AIDS tests the blood bank performed in February 1986 showed that he was positive for the AIDS antibody, but the blood bank did not disclose this vital information to him until seven months later. It was only after he had made another donation in August 1986 that the blood bank's director finally told him about his infection.

On August 16, 1987, nearly two years after the blood bank knew that they had provided the AIDS-contaminated blood to Gerald, they publicly perpetuated their deception about AIDS ever being transfused through their blood donors. In an article appearing in the *Spokesman-Review*, Spokane's daily newspaper, the blood bank's coordinator for donor acquirement said, "No AIDS-contaminated blood had ever been transfused into anyone in Spokane." This was a boldfaced lie because the blood bank had known of Gerald's infection since November 1985.

Regardless of their strategy for concealing vital information from Gerald, the donor, and the public, the blood bank has never explained why they waited so long to tell Gerald about his infection with the

AIDS virus. Their donor notification form for a donor whose blood reacted positively to the virus states the following:

DONORS WHOSE POSITIVE ELISA TESTS ARE CONFIRMED BY THE WESTERN BLOT SHOULD BE NOTIFIED WITHIN 55 DAYS.

Shortly after its discovery of Gerald's first confirmed AIDS test results, the blood bank made the connection between him and the donor of the contaminated unit, for in Gerald's blood-bank documents was the record of his transfusion at the hospital a year before. The donor was identified as another regular blood bank donor—the missing link in the chain had been established.

Notwithstanding this discovery, when the blood bank's director finally told Gerald about the test results nearly a year later, he said he did not know how Gerald could have become infected. This was another blatant lie. Rather than tell him the truth, the director implied that Gerald had engaged in some high-risk behavior such as homosexuality or prostitution, but when Gerald rolled up his pant leg and showed the surgical scar, the director was caught in his own web of deceit. Then he suggested Gerald not tell his wife. When Gerald said he would tell her the truth, the director then suggested he tell her it was chronic hepatitis. Again, Gerald refused to lie to Virginia.

Gerald immediately drove home. After his wife arrived there from a shopping trip, he met her in the driveway and asked her to come into the house. There he told her what he had just learned about his exposure to AIDS. For Virginia, "Hell opened up!" Despite this feeling, her job was to stand by her husband; they would fight the disease together.

Gerald's initial shock and devastation from the woefully belated disclosure of his infection changed to acute anger and humiliation. Why hadn't the blood bank, to which he had contributed so much during his lifetime, told him as soon as they knew? His anger was aggravated by the extreme anxiety of whether he had infected his wife, their family, friends, and the acquaintances with whom he had come into contact since he'd become infected. He also felt that had he known from the start, he would have taken better care of himself.

Even though Gerald and Virginia were committed to fighting his disease, Gerald was so humiliated by his infection that he could not even tell his children. Despite the shame, he expressed to his pastor how he felt about not learning of the infection sooner. Being a caring individual who was very concerned about hurting anyone else with his disease, he always made it a point to let people he met know that he carried the AIDS virus. This was particularly true when his pastor took him to his doctor's office or the hospital for tests and treatment. He told all healthcare workers about his disease so that they could decide for themselves whether they wanted to deal with him. If they did not, it was all right with him.

Gerald also told his pastor how upset he was by the blood bank's yearlong delay in notifying him of his infection. He constantly worried about whether he had infected others during the time that he hadn't known. Furthermore, he wondered about what had happened to the blood he had donated to the blood bank since his surgery. He quite rightly did not believe the blood bank's story that his blood had been destroyed. It was just one lie on top of another.

What was very frustrating for Gerald was that he donated five more units of blood after he had tested positive for the AIDS virus. Had the blood bank credited him for five units donated elsewhere when he asked their director to do so, he would never have given his blood to the blood bank after his surgery. Even though the director knew about Gerald's infection, he steadfastly refused to credit him because of the blood bank's policy against unsubstantiated donations elsewhere. Would that they had held to the truth so zealously, especially when they made deadly mistakes with their own donors. Even more outrageous than their endless cover-up was the blood bank's deliberate breach of their fiduciary duty to Gerald, i.e., their legal and moral obligation of trust to him.

There were times when people Gerald knew shunned him because of his infection. This hurt him very much. Even though he fought strenuously to save his life, he knew he was under a death sentence. It was just a matter of time before the disease would end his life.

Gerald's family suffered shock, devastation, anger, humiliation, and anxiety as well. The husband and father who had done so much for them began to waste away, physically, mentally, and emotionally. He and his wife could no longer plan anything and were forced to live day by day.

Because of her marriage vows, Virginia was totally committed to Gerald and never told him to leave the family home. While he did everything he could to protect others, she did everything she could to protect him. I firmly believe that she did. It is a marvelous tribute to their love for one another.

Immediately after finding out the terrible news, Gerald was seen by Dr. Daniel Coulston, a Spokane internist specializing in the treatment of AIDS patients. His examination and testing confirmed the HIV diagnosis. Gerald did everything Dr. Coulston prescribed, not only to save his life but also to protect his family and friends. The initial treatment was conservative because there was no medicine at that time to deal with his infection. He followed his physician's orders to the letter.

Even though he had, in the words of his wife, "lived to eat," Gerald watched his diet religiously, stopped drinking alcohol completely, and altered his lifestyle dramatically. He not only took sleeping pills and anti-depressants to deal with his anxiety but most important, also kept busy helping others. This was his nature.

In addition to his physician's treatment, Gerald's family, friends, and pastor provided the vital emotional support he desperately needed. His pastor ministered to him from the time Gerald first learned about his infection until the moment of his death. This was a great comfort and it helped him during his darkest hours.

Sadly but inevitably, the HIV infection destroyed Gerald's immune system. Now he was subject to substantially increased risk from opportunistic infection. This meant that he had no protection against whatever invader got into his body. Without any medicine or other treatment to combat this deficiency, his health deteriorated so much that he got full-blown AIDS.

Dr. Coulston then prescribed AZT, the only FDA-approved drug for the treatment of AIDS. Gerald started this therapy and he religiously followed other treatment. He even took ddI, an experimental drug for the treatment of AIDS, but since there was no cure for the disease, Dr. Coulston's early prognosis of death most regrettably proved true.

Gerald deteriorated rapidly after AIDS set in. The disease caused a lymphoma in his throat, which required surgery and radiation. The cancer and treatment made it virtually impossible for him to swallow anything but liquids, so he was eventually forced to take nutrition in fluid form. Just before he died, he could not even swallow water.

While recovering at home from his last hospitalization, Gerald began to bleed uncontrollably from his nose and mouth. Virginia called his pastor and asked him to take Gerald to the hospital. When the pastor arrived at their home, he was not allowed to come in until he put on latex gloves. They did not want Gerald's blood touching his pastor's unprotected hands. Once at the hospital, some of Gerald's blood spilled on the floor. He tried to clean it up so that one else would touch it.

To prevent his blood from spilling further, Gerald was asked to hold a bowl so that his blood would flow into it. He was in a seated position with the bowl cradled in his lap when his carotid artery ruptured. The pastor held his head as this was happening, but nothing could be done to stop the bleeding. Gerald mercifully died soon thereafter, still holding the bowl in his lap. The rupture was caused by erosion of the artery from the AIDS-related lymphoma. Tragically and ironically, no amount of blood could have saved Gerald's life.

As I write about this painful episode, several bad memories are dredged from the bottom of my mind like toxic heavy metals from the bottom of a badly polluted lake. I remember Gerald as a strong, robust man with big hands and wrists. He was born in Missouri, the "Show Me" state, and he typified this attitude. He was a man of action and few words. He did manual labor all his life and it showed, but when he shriveled away before my eyes, I found it very hard to see him. What I recall from this wasting was his watch. It was big, and it hung so loosely on his wrist from the toll of AIDS that it was unbearable for me to witness this dramatic deterioration. I had known him so long.

Furthermore, during the late 1980s, television coverage of Romanian infants showed the horrors these innocents suffered from

AIDS-contaminated blood transfusions. The anguish Gerald confided in me that his blood might have been put into their little bodies is indescribable. Then he bought a gun and told me he was seriously considering suicide. I believed him. I don't remember what I said to him when he told me this in my office. I knew the gun was in his truck parked outside. I have blotted my heartfelt advice out of my memory as to what convinced him not to do it, but I had never walked in his shoes. No other client, before or since, has ever told me about such contemplation. It is a heavy burden, and it is no wonder I have tried to exorcize these demons. Like toxic heavy metals, it is best to leave them undisturbed forever.

Chapter 10

The Failure of the Justice System

Law grinds the poor and rich men rule the law.
—Oliver Goldsmith

Gerald's case demanded an inordinate amount of time and energy. The litigation that ensued from his claim was both complex and expensive. Consequently, being a sole practitioner with no money to finance the costs, I associated two plaintiffs' personal injury lawyers, Bill Maxey of Maxey Law Offices in Spokane, a longtime friend and fellow Oregon Duck alum, and Paul Whelan of Stritmatter Kessler Whelan in Seattle, to help me prosecute the case against the hospital, the surgeon, the blood bank, and the anonymous donor.

The facts of Gerald's case proved beyond doubt that the blood bank was negligent as a matter of law. They caused his death and therefore his family was entitled to damages. The principal legal theory of recovery was that the blood bank was strictly liable for the harm caused to Gerald. This meant that by providing the AIDS-contaminated blood to him, whether for profit or not, the blood bank was at fault and should bear the consequences of the injury to Gerald rather than allowing such loss to fall upon him when he was entirely without fault. A Washington State Court of Appeals decision so held, thereby allowing the plaintiff to proceed on the claim that the nonprofit blood bank, which had supplied hepatitis-infected blood to her, was strictly liable. Therefore, all that is required of a plaintiff proceeding under the theory of strict liability is proof of his damages.

In addition to the foregoing facts and law supporting Gerald's case, we claimed that the blood bank was negligent in screening the donor and his blood for the AIDS virus. Our expert medical witnesses, one a dermatologist specializing in the treatment of AIDS patients and the other a Ph.D. specializing in epidemiology and public health, said this was the case. Since early 1983, it was well known by the medical and scientific community that HIV was blood borne. Surrogate testing was also available. This means that HIV can be detected in the blood with the hepatitis B core antibody test and the T-cell test. The blood bank did not use either of these tests before the adoption of the first FDA approved test ELISA—but they should have.

Furthermore, both of our expert witnesses said that not only was the blood bank negligent for failing to use surrogate tests on the donor's blood but also they improperly screened him at the time of the suspected donation. In particular, his elevated blood pressure indicated that he should not have donated blood on the day he did. More compelling was that the donor information sheet about AIDS purportedly given to him at that time did not provide adequate information, i.e., what kinds of high-risk behaviors, namely, homosexuality, bisexuality, and intravenous drug abuse, would preclude him from donating. Even if the blood bank had followed up with appropriate questioning of the donor, the medical questionnaire on the back side of his donor card with their questions and his answers about AIDS was "missing."

The significance of the "missing" questionnaire cannot be overstated. When the blood bank at last produced the donor's record of donation, only a photocopy of the front side with the donor's medical information was made for us; and pursuant to the trial court's order, to which I strenuously but uselessly objected and which was affirmed by the Washington State Supreme Court, the donor's name and any other identifying information were redacted. Regardless, the donor's original card was "lost" and only a facsimile of the back side with the standard, but unanswered, questionnaire was produced. His card was within the blood bank's exclusive control and it was absolutely imperative that it be maintained. Since it was not, the only conclusion that could be drawn was that whatever had been recorded on the back of the card would have been damning.

During the prosecution of the case, we were constantly battling "our worthy opponents" in their relentless motions, discovery, and other matters designed to delay the disposition of the litigation. Chief among the latter were two direct reviews by the Washington State Supreme Court of important pretrial rulings by the Spokane County Superior Court.

In the first Supreme Court case, we argued that the Washington State Court of Appeals decision, which allowed a plaintiff injured by hepatitis-contaminated blood provided by a nonprofit blood bank to pursue a claim of strict liability, entitled Gerald to seek recovery of damages via the same avenue of relief. The Court of Appeals held that a transaction involving the transfusion of blood supplied by a blood bank is the sale of a defective product, not the provision of a service.

In overruling the Court of Appeals, the Supreme Court said that provision of blood constitutes a service, not a sale of a defective product. Consequently, claims based upon strict liability would not be permitted against providers of blood for any reason. This left us with only one basis of liability: negligence. Therefore, we had to prove fault as well as damages. The effect of the Supreme Court's ruling made it much more difficult for us to succeed.

Following the Supreme Court decision, Joanne Werner, then a University of Puget Sound Law School graduate and now a plaintiffs' attorney, asked me to review her proposed law review article, "An Argument for Removing the Statutory Shield from HIV-Infected Blood." It criticized the court's ruling that blood banks are immune from strict liability because in a case such as ours, we were faced with the complicated, if not impossible, task of obtaining sufficient proof to establish a negligence case. Chief among them were the problems of inconsistency of screening standards of donors and inability to access information about them. Two years earlier I had sent Joanne the pleadings in the case, which she used to craft her argument. I checked her facts, made minor corrections, and then returned her draft. Even though her law school professors urged her to have the article published, the law review board refused to do it. To this day it remains unpublished, but not so for other critical law reviews and periodicals, particularly *The Journal of Pharmacy & Law,* "Comment: Culpable Conduct with Impunity: The Blood Industry and the FDA's Responsibility for the Spread of AIDS Through Blood Products" (3 J. Pharmacy & Law 129, 1994). Specifically, blood is a product. Thus it is clearly erroneous for courts to conclude that providing blood is not a sale but a service because patients in the hospital are charged a separate fee for the blood they use.

Chapter 11

The Settlement

Some justice is better than none at all.
—Claudius

It had been more than six long, arduous years. Gerald was dead from AIDS and the next step was a jury trial. The costs to this point were $60,000, and the estimated trial costs were another $50,000. His widow, Virginia, was worn out, so after a daylong mediation we settled for the policy limits of the blood bank's liability insurance policy. Since the settlement was confidential, the amount could not be disclosed. Regardless, at the end of my mediation letter, I summed up:

> It is clearly evident that the blood bank is liable for the injuries and damages caused to our client and his family. They must be compensated not only because the blood bank was negligent in screening the donor and his blood, but also because they tried to hide the truth from the family when they first learned about our client's infection. This egregious conduct cannot go unsanctioned.
>
> What makes the case of the family so important is that the blood bank, as a healthcare provider, has a legal duty to protect the public health. Our client was a man who time and again responded to the blood bank's call for his blood. If the blood bank's outrageous mistreatment of him is standard operating procedure, what will it be toward other AIDS transfusion victims who have done little or nothing for the blood bank? They must

be held accountable for their unlawful misconduct, especially when they ask the public to donate blood. In light of this, the damages that the family ask for are the only way to compensate them for the reprehensible behavior of the blood bank, especially when our client did so much for the blood bank.

A couple of legal aphorisms came into play for our Gerald and Virginia's case:
Justice delayed is justice denied.
A poor settlement is better than a good lawsuit.

Indeed, the appellate process had not only delayed justice but the Supreme Court had also denied it to our clients. The surgeon, the hospital, and the blood bank were all well heeled and their lawyers well paid. There was no incentive for the blood bank to settle until they were the only defendant left to stand trial. Then and only then did they capitulate, but the toll for our clients was unbelievably heavy. It was burdensome for their legal counsel as well. For Bill and Paul, they were on the hook for absorbing the exorbitant costs because Gerald and Virginia could never pay them, and for me, the physical and emotional toll, especially of dealing personally with the couple, left me exhausted and bitter. They were such decent human beings that at times I wanted to give up and end their legal nightmare with any kind of recovery, but I persevered, so in the end, the poor settlement Bill, Paul, and I mediated was better than the good lawsuit. Some justice and some money are better than none at all!

Chapter 12

The Aftermath

Oh, what a tangled web we weave when first we practice to deceive.
—Walter Scott

In the fall of 1989, the Spokane County Superior Court dismissed Gerald and Virginia's complaint against the blood donor with prejudice. The donor was still alive then. Try as we might, the trial court would not allow us to learn his identity. Based upon severely circumscribed discovery, we were forced to rely solely on his testimony, his wife's, the blood bank's records, and the records of his healthcare providers that he was not a homosexual, bisexual, or intravenous drug abuser. Without his identity we could not find out from independent sources whether he was telling the truth about not being a high-risk donor. Consequently, we appealed the trial court's order of dismissal.

In the second direct review of a pretrial ruling, the Supreme Court consolidated our case with a King County case involving the same issue, namely, whether the identity of an anonymous donor infected with HIV/AIDS was discoverable. Therefore, both were argued at the same time. The court, however, bifurcated the two cases after oral argument, and issued its decisions separately. The reason for doing this, without giving us the option to object to bifurcation, was simple: They couldn't be reconciled because they were logically inconsistent.

By the time of the Supreme Court's decisions, Gerald was dead, but the donor was alive. In the King County case, however, both the plaintiff and the donor were dead. This was the only material difference between the two cases. In our case the Supreme Court denied us discovery of the donor's identity because we couldn't establish that he was not credible. In the King County case, the Supreme Court allowed the plaintiff discovery of the donor's identity. Just as in our first case against the blood bank, the Supreme Court protected the donor at the expense of our clients.

Nonetheless, we discovered his identity when an anonymous source telephoned and gave the name of the donor and his occupation. Furthermore, he said that the donor was a member of a high-risk group. Armed with this tip, we promptly moved to reopen the case against him. This is what we learned about the donor:

♦ He lied and he deceived his wife.

♦ He was homosexual and bisexual.

♦ He died of AIDS.

Despite all this evidence, the courts refused to let us reopen the case. It was a mockery of our clients and a failure of the justice system. The deceit of the blood bank and the donor made our task extremely onerous. And the justice system enabled them to perpetrate their lies with impunity. By so doing, it materially prejudiced Gerald and Virginia who were good and decent human beings. The tangled web the blood bank and the donor wove caused the premature deaths of our clients.

When I sum up what Gerald, through the sacrifice of his life, and Bill, Paul, and I, by dint of our effort, did, it comes to this: Together we made the blood supply safer for this country. The blood-banking industry is asking the hard questions now that they did not ask, but should have, when the donor gave his blood. In the Inland Northwest Blood Center's Donor Education Materials, there are very blunt descriptions of what "sexual contact" is and how HIV/AIDS is spread through such contact. The message is clear: Do not give if the donor fits the description of this high-risk behavior.

I owe a debt of gratitude to Merri Hartse, the electronic resources librarian of Gonzaga University Law School. When I heard from Joanne Werner in January 2015 that her article had never been published, I was dejected. No one knew, I thought, what she and I knew. When we at last finished Gerald and Virginia's case in 1993, I put it out of my mind. It was too raw and painful to contemplate. I wanted desperately to move on, so for more than two decades it lay underground like the cicada. Then Merri helped me research my Supreme Court cases online. It was an epiphany! All three have been cited more than 700 times by subsequent courts, law reviews, periodicals, treatises, briefs, and motions, some of which have been critical of the Supreme Court's decisions. At last I felt vindicated.

Chapter 13

My Own Odyssey

You are a hard man, Odysseus, never downhearted and never tired!
You must be made of iron!
—Homer

When I started on my own odyssey with Gerald in 1986, I was thirty-nine years old. My JRA seemed to be under control at that time. In fact, with my brother's encouragement and support, I had already participated as the 1,500-meter swimmer in my first triathlon, the Lake Coeur d'Alene Scenic Challenge, the year before. I would continue this endeavor the next three years, from 1986 until 1988. Then I stopped. On reflection I now know why.

The burden of my voyage in the unending storms the justice system hurled at Gerald and me, like the wrath of Poseidon at Odysseus, was compounded by two other important factors. The first factor was dealing with Gerald. The drugs prescribed for his treatment did not stem the HIV onslaught on his immune system. He was dying before my eyes.

Like Gerald's drug treatment for his HIV, the prescription for my JRA did not stop its attack on my immune system. This was the other factor that pressed down on me during my seven-year representation of this decent, hardworking man. Although he was the primary focus of my practice from 1986 until 1993, I still handled matters for other clients, and, as my children grew, I became more involved in their lives. The stress arising from my commitments to all of these relationships wore me down. The roller-coaster ride I could never get off inevitably led to a steep and dangerous downward spiral.

The first symptoms of this course surfaced in early 1988. Despite holding my own with various therapies for my fingers, wrists, knees, ankles, and feet, I began suffering stiffness and pain in my neck, jaw, shoulders, hips, ribs, and right elbow. The balls of both feet were hurting too, with curling of several of my toes. Most important of all, my right thumb was permanently bent outward at the first joint from the nail. The cause of this deformity was the repetitive use of my dictation equipment. Consequently, I underwent joint fusion therapy right after my fourth Lake Coeur d'Alene Triathlon, but before the surgeon operated, I told him I would not consent to a blood transfusion if needed during my surgery or hospital stay.

Since I had donated a couple of units for the wounded Vietnam War soldiers during my UW years, I told my surgeon I could either self-donate through the autologous procedure or have my father, also an experienced blood donor with the same blood type, have his drawn and stored in advance. Again and again he answered the call for our neighbor's son. Born with hemophilia, many of his childhood injuries required blood transfusions. When my father was home from his travels during these terrible times, he, just like Gerald, always helped. My good father donated, time and again to the blood bank, not only to help not our neighbors' son but also to help other people he didn't even know. Because the surgeon said the risk of blood loss requiring a transfusion was so low for my operation, however, undertaking these precautions was unnecessary. This surgery, as well as the previous synovectomy on the big knuckles of my left hand, limited my manual dexterity even more.

Unlike the wily Odysseus whose resourcefulness and cunning enabled him to defeat his enemies time and again, my enemy is insidious and waging war twenty-four hours a day, 365 days a year. JRA is relentless and will not be beaten until the cure for it is found. Consequently, my heart drifted downward during my odyssey and I was tiring more and more. In this dark time of my life, my will of iron began to fail.

Chapter 14

Death of a Friend

The sun for sorrow shall not show its head.
—William Shakespeare

The sorrow Shakespeare wrote of in *Romeo and Juliet* was the kind arising from unexpected death. I knew Gerald was dying and this inevitable fact weighed heavily on me, but his death in August 1990 did not affect me nearly so much as the unexpected death of my best friend, Paul, less than three months later. A head-on car crash claimed his life. He was just forty-three years old, leaving behind his father, Leslie, his sisters, Kathleen and Maureen, his wife, Stephanie, and their four young daughters, Melissa, Molly, Shannon, and Allyson. Paul's mother, Edith, had predeceased him in 1977.

Paul and I met in the fourth grade at St. Augustine's Parochial School. It was the first and last class we shared together, from parochial school through college. I think this fact is one of the reasons we were lifelong friends. By this I mean we were not constantly present together in the same schoolroom. Thus it was easier to remain friends. Several of the ways we did this was by playing together in Manito Park, also less than a block from his home. We would practice hitting baseballs to each other and throwing them back and forth. There were the sleepovers at each other's homes. Many a time they led to wrestling matches, which resulted in our parents' separating us, sometimes for the night. We were each other's best man. If ever there was a true friend, it was Paul. His visiting me every day during my childhood convalescence when he was only twelve years old was a testament to his character and commitment.

During our thirty-one-year relationship, Paul and I shared many experiences, but they naturally grew scarcer as we grew older. Our marriages, families, and careers created this scarcity. Nevertheless, they made us appreciate life and helped in developing our pragmatic, yet sometimes skeptical, even cynical view of the world. Our droll sense of humor played a major role in our development. Proof of this was our mutual appreciation of the witty cartoons featured in *The Far Side.* As a matter of fact, during my last visit with Paul in the summer of 1990, he told me he had arranged with Gary Larson, creator of *The Far Side,* for a donation of one of his original cartoons to a charitable auction.

We also shared a keen interest in the Rolling Stones. It was natural, I can attest to that. Paul's appreciation for music matured with his drumming. Many a time Vivian and I would watch him play at his band's gigs, whether it was rock & roll or country & western. It was pure, unadulterated fun. Even though we will not have the great good fortune of listening to Paul drum on his Ludwig kit in this life, the spirit of his drumming lives on. Paul's father gave the kit to my nephew, Mike, who was just learning how to play the drums. Although he cut his teeth on Beatles songs, Mike has subconsciously been imbued with the beat of the far superior rhythm Charlie Watts instilled in the kit through Paul. He recognized great drumming talent when he heard it, whether the Stones' drummer played R&B, C&W, or R&R. Once Mike could afford his own kit, he returned Paul's drums to his daughters. Molly's husband, Bryan, restored them beautifully. The distinctive Ludwig logo emblazoned on the big bass drum brings back the fond memories I have of this good and decent man, affectionately known to his coterie of friends and Stones' fans as Finkle.

While Mike will never admit to me that the Stones are the greatest band ever, I know he will recant by commencing my good ol' Irish wake, on Paul's kit, with *Start Me Up.* Then, for the benefit of his Lithuanian mother, my dear sister-in-law, affectionately known as Aunt Val, he shall pound out the perfect beat for the loose and lusty

Honky Tonk Woman, then the sweet and saucy *Brown Sugar,* and finally the crossfire hurricane *Jumpin' Jack Flash.* It'll be a gas, gas, gas!

Unlike me, Paul did not suffer from any apparent disability. If he did, stoic that he was, he never told me, but his late sister, Kathleen, did suffer from a disability for her entire life. She was born with Down syndrome. Paul thus understood disability quite well and what it meant for me. His parents taught him how to help his sister navigate the daily trials and tribulations her life presented. The lessons he learned from this experience led to a lifetime of helping less fortunate individuals. Before his death, he was very active with the Big Brothers & Big Sisters, the United Way, and the ARC. His service was particularly noteworthy because he worked one-to-one with developmentally disabled individuals like his sister.

In my eulogy at Paul's funeral service I highlighted his qualities of kindness and compassion for the disabled because I had been a direct beneficiary of these attributes. I concluded my remembrances by saying that what would sustain me during the dark days ahead was how Paul had helped me, time and again, deal with my disability and how he had helped so many others deal with theirs. The best way he did this for me was to never let me use it as an excuse. When we mixed it up through wrestling, he didn't hold back. Neither did I. This was how "baby boomer boys" settled their differences when oral argument was useless, and we usually ended up worn out and ready to move on to the next challenge.

What I did not foresee at Paul's funeral service is that I would follow his example of kindness and compassion for the disabled in the years to come. During the interim, the sorrow I would suffer was different from the kind brought on by my best friend's unexpected death. It was a long, drawn-out lament. As my health faded, my darkness grew.

Chapter 15

Trial and Error

Our deeds determine us, as much as we determine our deeds.
—George Eliot

Because of the pain and stiffness that was affecting more and more of my body, I either supplemented or supplanted my non-steroidal anti-inflammatory drugs (NSAIDs) with a regimen of other anti-inflammatory prescription medicines. They consisted of corticosteroids, cox-2 inhibitors, antibiotics, and disease-modifying anti-rheumatic drugs (DMARDs). One of these medications, injectable methotrexate, was especially hard on me. Not only did the weekly shots lay me up in bed for an entire day but, due to its major potential for liver toxicity, I was also strictly forbidden to consume alcoholic beverages. Being an aficionado of Scotch whisky, this prohibition added palpably to my anguish.

Regardless, when one drug didn't work, I tried another, but just like the NSAIDs, each had side effects too numerous to list. Suffice to say that in conjunction with the rheumatoid arthritis they've produced problems for my heart, lungs, kidneys, and liver, but with these organs hidden from view and not then needing treatment, my immediate concern was the evident adverse effect of the never-ending inflammation of my joints. During this period, most, if not all of its signs and symptoms—pain, swelling, redness, and heat—plagued me incessantly. One of the consequences I vividly remember was the inflammation of the knees. It became so severe at times that my rheumatologists would first draw off the accumulated fluid with a large hypodermic needle and then inject my knees with cortisone. One treating physician even advised me to undergo synovectomies of both knees, but based on prior experience with this surgery on my left hand, I refused to follow his suggestion. I chose to hobble in pain rather than lose even more range of motion.

One of the results of a prolonged battle with rheumatoid arthritis is that the inflammatory response of this autoimmune disease erodes the bones at the joints. Orthopedic evaluations and periodic x-rays confirmed that I was experiencing this erosion, especially in my wrists, fingers, ankles, and toes. Consequently, in 1991 and 1994 I underwent additional joint-fusion surgery for hammertoe correction on both feet. What wasn't so evident from the unchecked nature of the disease and the lengthy corticosteroid treatment for it was the effect on the rest of my skeleton. Both can hasten bone loss. Despite my exercise routine and a large daily dosage of calcium supplements, a bone mineral density screening in 1997 disclosed I was severely osteoporotic. Placed on yet another prescription drug with its own set of side effects, I now confronted the risk of fracture.

A perfect storm was beginning to form. The stress of yet another diagnosis and the mounting fatigue from my daily struggles were wearing me down. Although I have not lost faith in some forms of allopathic treatment, i.e., Western medications used by American mainstream doctors and hospitals, over time I have relied significantly relied less on chemical drugs and have incorporated more complementary remedies into my life.

The first complementary therapy I use each day is hydrotherapy. It has been a major component of my healthcare regimen since 1978. I have also employed acupuncture and diet changes, and with the knowledge and support of Dr. Jon Stevenson, a competent, caring, and compassionate physician and my rheumatologist from 1993 until his retirement, I use naturopathic remedies, principally herbs and supplements.

Even with daily doses of a DMARD, a corticosteroid, and an NSAID, the naturopathic course of treatment prescribed by physicians and naturopaths had failed to stem the increasing ill effects of my arthritis. It was winning and I was losing, but I still refused to yield.

After I opened my law office in 1978, my interest in finding a better way to control and maybe even cure my arthritis picked up steam. In addition to borrowing materials from the local libraries and surfing the Internet, I maintained a record of newspaper and magazine articles featuring various remedies. Whether allopathic or complementary, I was willing to incorporate the safe and effective ones into my treatment. In particular, if the allopathic pharmaceutical drugs specifically developed for rheumatoid arthritis received the FDA stamp of approval as "safe and effective," I would discuss their potential application with my rheumatologists. I also explored with them my volunteering for a clinical trial. My motivation to be a "guinea pig" was not, however, altruistic. All I wanted was to be healthy again.

In 1990 a Japanese research institute was testing an anti-rejection drug, called FK506, at the University of Pittsburgh Medical Center. I learned about it at that time from an article in the lay press. It was quite successful in preventing liver transplant rejection. Derived from a soil fungus, it inhibited the action of white blood cells thought to be a cause of inflammation. The scientists testing the drug planned on investigating its potential for treating rheumatoid arthritis.

It wasn't until late 1997 that the stars aligned for me to enroll in a randomized, double blind, placebo-controlled, dose-finding clinical trial of FK 506. This meant that I was to receive either a placebo or one of three different dosing regimens of the drug. I was also to be assigned to one of the treatment regimens by chance, and neither Dr. Stevenson nor I was to know what regimen I was taking. The purpose of the study was to test the effectiveness, safety, and best dose of the drug in rheumatoid arthritis patients who could not tolerate methotrexate. As my trial progressed at Arthritis Northwest, my initial optimism ebbed. I could neither feel nor see any improvement. Once the six-month study concluded, I was informed I had received the lowest dosage of the drug.

Notwithstanding this failure, Dr. Stevenson recommended a new DMARD. He had recently injected my knees with cortisone, but they continued to bother me. In a letter to him in March 1999, I told him that I suspected the new drug was not going to work, but my hope had not yet faded away. I closed my letter with a request for a recent medical journal article detailing the results of a new type of medicine, a biologic response modifier (BRM) called Etanercept. According to all measures of disease activity, the addition of this drug to the methotrexate therapy for rheumatoid arthritis patients in the control groups showed marked improvement. What stopped me from starting Etanercept, however, was the methotrexate. Consequently, I continued with the new DMARD, which, like methotrexate, is toxic to the liver.

Chapter 16

Crisis

Home is the sailor, home from the sea
And the hunter home from the hill.
—Robert Louis Stevenson

I first read Stevenson's famous stanza at the funeral service of a young man I knew from grade school. He was a talented individual whose life was cut short because of the deep depression he had suffered. His death still impacts me when I hear the sorrowful words of Stevenson's dirge.

In 1999, I hoped I would be home from the sea, home from the hill. Without a new treatment, I could not save my life. Just as Gerald had experienced, my will to live wavered. Though I did not contemplate suicide like he had, I thought it was just a matter of time before death would claim me. Such was my mental state that I even began believing my JRA was a precursor to cancer. If I could have then traded my condition for the risk of facing violent injury or death in the Vietnam War three decades earlier, I would have. I was that desperate, that despondent.

My desperation and my despondency were so overwhelming that I didn't realize what effects they were having on my children. In a poignant letter to me from Matt, written on the eve of my fifty-second birthday, I learned how he felt about living with a disabled father. Matt began by thanking me for, as Lincoln said to Grant, Sherman, and Porter about what to do with the South just before the Civil War ended, "letting him up easy" after several of his youthful escapades.

He then noted my health was worsening. Specifically, he said I had lost a lot of weight. What worried him the most, though, was that I worked only four hours a day and usually went right to bed when I got home. He then concluded his letter by saying, "I wish you a wonderful birthday and I hope you start feeling better. I love you, Dad." Matt's sympathy touched me deeply. Eight years later his emotion evolved into empathy. On Vivian's fifty-eighth birthday, Matt suffered a horrible injury to his left hand. After a lengthy rehabilitation, he regained most of its function, but occasionally he feels arthritis in his fingers from cold temperatures or strenuous activity. He now knows personally what this condition means.

Monica has expressed similar sentiments in many of her notes and letters to me, and she has told others about the effect my rheumatoid arthritis has had on her. What she said touched me as deeply as her brother's letter did.

Being the children of a chronically ill father, Monica and Matt must certainly have wondered at times during their childhood why the wheel of fate had spun them such a parent. The ups and downs of their own lives then were enough to contend with. While they were growing up, one of my biggest concerns for them was their health. I sometimes felt like a hawk, watching for any signs and symptoms of illness, particularly strep throat, which might trigger the beginning of a life with rheumatoid arthritis. There is a genetic component to this condition and a history of it in my mother's family. I feel the same way about my wonderful grandchildren, Corinne, Lauren, and Ryan, but whether through the vigilance of Vivian and me, our children's lifestyles, plain good luck, or other factors too numerous to even speculate upon, Monica and Matt have been blessed with good health, and so have our dear granddaughters and grandson. May it always continue!

In the fall of 1999, Matt commenced his college education with a business curriculum at Western Washington University. Monica, who had started there in 1997, was at the University of Maine on a one-year exchange program. Just as I had done during my undergraduate stint, her principal studies were chemistry. After a two-week family vacation in northern New England, Vivian, Matt, and I left Monica at the Orono campus and returned home. A month later I took Matt and his belongings to Bellingham, Washington. Once he was settled in his dormitory, I left for Spokane. It was a difficult departure for me because our nest was now empty. To be sure there would be the winter, spring, and summer breaks, but our son had joined our daughter on the path to independent living. This was what Vivian and I wanted for both of them, but realization of the goal had its bittersweet moments for us.

Nonetheless, my path was fast leading to a crossroads. Shortly after Matt had written his letter, my knees once again swelled so much that Dr. Stevenson had to inject them yet again with cortisone. He was a master at applying this temporary relief. I remember the very last time I ever had to go through that terrifying experience. With steady eye and pinpoint accuracy, he expertly marked with his pen the precise point of entry and gently, painlessly, injected the needle. He then drew off the fluid and drove home the drug. Mission Not Only Possible—Mission Accomplished! Instead of being wheel-chaired out of his office, I walked with Vivian to our car and went home.

Chapter 17

The Hand of Fate Is on Me Now

I look inside myself and see my heart is black.
I see my red door I must have it painted black.
Maybe then I'll fade away and not have to face the facts.
It's not easy facing up when your whole world is black.
—Mick Jagger and Keith Richards

As my darkness grew, I genuinely believed my world would soon be "black as night, black as coal," but because I am genetically wired stubborn Irish, I steadfastly refused to yield to my nemesis. In late 1991, I had read an article about clinical trials of a drug developed for rheumatoid arthritis by Immunex, a research and development company headquartered in Seattle. They were going to conduct their trials at Northwestern University Medical School in Chicago. Scheduled to start in March 1992, the first protocol in the studies would evaluate intra-articular injections of the unnamed drug into the inflamed, swollen knee joints of "human guinea pigs." The second study would evaluate daily subcutaneous injections of the drug for twenty-eight days. It was set to begin in the spring of 1992. After reviewing the first study's inclusion and exclusion criteria, provided to me by Immunex's assistant director of clinical affairs, I decided I wouldn't meet the eligibility requirements, but I filed the documentation with my other arthritis research materials nonetheless.

Then, in late 1996, I read a story in the local newspaper about Lindagail Dixon, a forty-two-year-old woman who had participated in the Immunex trials of three drugs. Diagnosed with rheumatoid arthritis at the age of twenty-five and a single mother of four children, Lindagail and thirty other patients were being tested with one of the unnamed drugs for three months by Dr. Scott Baumgartner, the father of one of Monica's friends. It was yet another memorable, ironic episode in my life with JRA.

Regardless, before enrollment Lindagail had repeatedly waxed and waned between remissions and flares. Like many a rheumatoid arthritis patient, she was at the end of her rope. At times she couldn't hold her cross-stitch needle or zip up her clothes. Even stirring a pot of soup was painful, but she bit the bullet and started the drug. Almost immediately after her first injection, she went running. I then called her.

Nearly 800 patients nationwide had taken part in the three studies of the new but still unnamed drugs. Most of the patients reported improvements in their swollen joints, often within two weeks. Dr. Baumgartner administered different levels of the drug or a placebo to his enrolled patients, all of whom had failed to respond to traditional therapy. The Spokane test site attracted more patients than any of the other test sites. In Dr. Baumgartner's opinion, what accounted for such local participation was the large rheumatology practice and number of patients willing to try new treatments. Regrettably, I wasn't one of them; as Immunex had conducted the studies, I figured I wouldn't have been eligible. In any event I filed the article with the rest of my arthritis research materials and plodded on.

A year later another article appeared in the local newspaper about the Immunex studies. The results from the Phase 3 testing—the last stage required before the data could be submitted to the FDA—had just been released. They were promising. The new drug, named Enbrel, was so effective in the treatment of rheumatoid arthritis that even rheumatologists were excited. Dr. Baumgartner said that since starting his rheumatology practice in 1980, there had been, until now, basically nothing new. Lindagail, single mother of four children, had improved to such an extent in her three-year treatment with Enbrel that she had gone from being a sedentary secretary to an energetic restaurant manager on her feet ten hours a day.

Enbrel was approved for public use in 1998, but even with my knowledge of its development since 1991, I was not yet using the "miracle drug." Although my weight had stabilized by December 1999, my joints were still stiff and sore, especially in my wrists and hands, every time I woke up from restless sleep. Loss of it was made up during the day by continuing my reduced office time to four hours. I could not keep this up much longer.

Chapter 18

The Horns of a Dilemma

When you come to a fork in the road, take it.
—Yogi Berra

The comical malapropism of famous major league baseball catcher Yogi Berra appropriately described my predicament at the end of 1999. By then I was eligible to use Enbrel; however, several factors halted me at the fork. The drug is self-administered through weekly subcutaneous injections.

Ever since my mother's periodic immunizations of my siblings and me against various childhood diseases with her reusable needle, made duller still by my brother's elephantine skin, and my pediatric physician's routine blood draws with a similar instrument following the onset of rheumatic fever, I have been loath to suffer intentional punctures of my circulatory system. With my small, deep-seated veins, there have been many times when phlebotomists would not strike red, even after many painful pokes. I genuinely felt sorry for them when they couldn't get what every good vampire worth her salt desperately seeks.

My reluctance to self-inject Enbrel on this account was not the stumbling block. The injections can cause site reactions, such as redness, itching, pain, and swelling. The risk Enbrel creates for infections increases because, just like other toxic rheumatoid arthritis drugs, it suppresses the immune system. Sepsis, better known as blood poisoning, is also a threat. Added to these terrors is lymphoma, cancer of the lymphatic system, and a visit by the Grim Reaper is a distinct possibility, but what made me pause is the warning on the label that seven new malignancies were observed in the clinical trial patients for up to eighteen months. When the millennium arrived, however, my vacillation ceased. Knowing that I had explored every alternative, I followed Berra's advice and took the fork in the road.

After consulting with Dr. Stevenson and my family, I girded up my loins for an Enbrel experiment. I remember in particular talking with Matt about my feelings before commencing. Typically, he didn't say much. Even though he thought it was my call, I believe he wanted me to try the drug. His letter of the previous July was the basis for that belief. I also spoke a couple of times with Lindagail Dixon who had been featured in the press as one of the Spokane Enbrel "guinea pigs." Her positive four-year experience was additional grist for my mill. Overcoming my anxieties about self-injection and the possible adverse reactions, I at last took the plunge, literally and figuratively, on March 1, 2000.

By embarking on the Enbrel path, I had not thrown caution to the wind. In my youth, my parents had nicknames for my siblings and me. Being a second child, I learned from my brother's experiences that certain behavior was just too risky to emulate. If it involved an element of danger, I was even more circumspect, but when I failed to follow my instincts for self-preservation and engaged in activities potentially hazardous to my health, I tried to take precautions. So it was that my parents aptly nicknamed me Cautious John.

There were many occasions that justified calling me by this moniker, but what I remember as the best evidence for my parents' declaration was my infrequent ascents to and descents from the top of the Ponderosa pine in our backyard. Whereas my brother and sister scampered up and down this hundred-foot tree like lemurs, I inched up its trunk like a sloth. I carefully inspected every limb, above or below me, that I would cling to next, and it took a long time to finish this task. Thus my pitiful performance in climbing the tree, as my parents put it, "with one foot on the ground," was proof positive that I deserved their apt nickname.

It is not to say, however, that I approached every risky situation so cautiously. In my pre-JRA days I was very fond of taking down larger opponents in tackle football, whether at the practices or during the games. I also enjoyed the occasional wrestling match in which angry moments led to body blows with clenched fists, and I didn't always escape these endeavors free of bruises or loss of blood, but whether consciously or not, I usually weighed the risks of success or failure before engaging in such activities.

Even after JRA became a permanent companion, I did not refrain from engaging in dangerous sports. Many is the time I stared down steep ski slopes and thought it would be crazy to rely on two skinny slats for getting me to the bottom of the run. Nevertheless, I pointed them in that direction and took off, reaching speeds calculated to result in broken bones or torn tendons at the slightest miscue. Also, scuba-diving adventures, particularly off the Pacific Coast of Mexico, produced occasional panic at depth. A close encounter with a rather large moray eel whose gaping mouth and needle teeth temporarily took my breath away is still a vivid memory of risky behavior I voluntarily undertook.

There were other instances of derring-do that irrefutably demonstrated the temporary but total loss of a sound and disposing mind. Suffice to say that most of these experiences were in the premarital phase of my life. After our children arrived on the scene, these exploits became fewer and farther between, but once Monica and Matt were safely ensconced in college, I took on the biggest challenge of my life: starting on the Enbrel injections.

Following the first shot at Dr. Stevenson's office, I was on my own. Overcoming the psychological barrier of self-injection was the hardest part. It took a while to do this, but my commitment to this course of treatment was resolute. Once I mastered the technique, the side effect of injection site reaction disappeared, and after just one month, I noticed a significant improvement in my arthritis.

As 2000 rolled to its conclusion, other changes in my health practices showed their beneficial effects too. I started a physical therapy program at St. Luke's Rehabilitation Institute in Spokane. Their staff, equipment, and facilities, especially their wonderfully soothing warm-water pool, provided physical therapy benefits for my body, and in addition to my regular lap swimming, I resumed a weight lifting program there that I had learned in 1996. Enbrel was in its post-marketing phase, the adverse event surveillance system run by the FDA. I questioned whether the drug would be safe over the long term, and the adverse reactions observed during the clinical trials, particularly malignancies, were never far from my mind. I still continued to ask Dr. Stevenson about alternative treatments and even a reduction in my dosage of Enbrel, but there was nothing else for me on the horizon. Moreover, a short-term lowering in and lengthening of the amount and period between shots stalled my progress, so I returned to the normal dosing of what was looking more to be the "miracle drug" I had long awaited.

Thus, after being denied admission to the ranks of participants in the clinical trials because of ineligibility, and continuing to endure untold suffering and limiting of activity, I finally had found a source of significant relief. My hope and persistence were paying off.

Chapter 19

Be It Resolved

To improve lives through leadership in the prevention, control, and cure of arthritis.
—Arthritis Foundation Mission Statement

My first active involvement with the Arthritis Foundation began in February 2001. I had known about this patient-oriented, nonprofit organization long before then because I had subscribed to their periodical, *Arthritis Today*, and had purchased some of their publications dealing with rheumatoid arthritis. Feeling much improved in early 2001 because of the health regimen I was practicing, I knew from my lengthy history with arthritis that unless a cure was discovered, I, and millions of Americans like me, could not escape its grip. Since part of the foundation's mission is devoted to finding a cure, I resolved to help them the best way I could: advocacy.

At the time I set upon the course of becoming a foundation advocate, I had been practicing law for twenty-three years. During that time I sharpened my writing and speaking skills through representation of many different clients in many different forums, but as a sole practitioner, my professional obligation was usually to an individual, not to an organization. As the new decade evolved, however, so did my role as a "mouthpiece." I had begun the transition from private paladin to public advocate.

My first foray into the world of volunteer advocacy for the foundation was contacting my Congressional representative, George Nethercutt. Before his election, he had been a fellow Spokane lawyer and had worked for Judge Williams while attending Gonzaga Law School. We also had a mutual interest in chronic childhood conditions. His daughter had contracted juvenile diabetes at a young age and was thus dependent upon self-injections of insulin. On behalf of the foundation I was seeking his support for a bill pending in Congress that would provide Medicare coverage of innovative, self-injectable biologic therapies such as Enbrel for chronic diseases. He gave it willingly.

The next step in the arena of public advocacy was training at the foundation's annual Advocacy Summit in Washington, D.C. Entitled "Together Making A Difference," the three-day session convened on February 25, 2001. More than 140 delegates from across the country learned about the important issues directly impacting the quality of their lives and the lives of millions of other Americans afflicted with arthritis. After two days' preparation, we and foundation staff met with members of Congress, told our individual stories, and asked for support of, among other important matters, Medicare coverage of self-injected biologics.

In early May 2001, I returned to Washington and met Senator Patty Murray, a Democratic colleague of our state's other senator, Maria Cantwell, and principal sponsor of a bill to amend the Social Security Act. The purpose of the bill was Medicare coverage of self-injected biologics such as Enbrel. I later met Congresswoman Jennifer Dunn, a Republican representing Bellevue, Washington, constituents. She was the principal sponsor in the House of Representatives of the same bill Senator Murray had introduced. In telling my story to each of them, I learned that their mothers had suffered with arthritis—one rheumatoid and the other osteoarthritis. With the sponsorship of Senator Murray and Congresswoman Dunn, along with the significant bipartisan support they had garnered from their congressional colleagues, I thought that the thirty-word amendment to the Social Security Act, to become effective on January 1, 2002, was "just a shot away."

Chapter 20

That Terrible Day:
September 11, 2001

Oh, a storm is threat'ning my very life today.
If I don't get some shelter, o yeah, I'm gonna fade away.
—Mick Jagger and Keith Richards

On September 10, 2001, I headed east once again via Seattle. There I met Janet Widmyer, a young mother with JRA whom the foundation had asked me to escort to Washington, D.C., for an important meeting. Janet was from Alaska and it was her first trip to our nation's capital. Like me she had started Enbrel. Our flight stopped at the Minneapolis-St. Paul airport where we nearly missed the connecting jet to D.C. In fact, the aircraft door had been closed. It was only at my insistence that it was opened and we were allowed on board. After the next day, airlines would never again accede to this type of demand.

Our mission seemed simple enough. We were part of a gathering of eighteen foundation delegates from around the country, all with arthritis and beneficiaries of self-injected biologics, who would participate in the foundation's advocacy program, "Access to Innovative Therapies: Arthritis and Medicare." As part of their commitment to ensuring that all Americans have access to therapies they need to treat and prevent disease, the foundation had issued a position statement on prescription drugs for Medicare beneficiaries. A key element of the statement focused on ensuring that they have access to the newer biologics which improve the lives of arthritis patients. The delegates' role in implementing this policy was to tell their stories to members of Congress following a breakfast with Senator Murray and Congresswoman Dunn, the sponsors of the bills expanding Medicare coverage of certain self-injected biologics, on September 12.

As Janet and I sat at breakfast on September 11, Fred Price, the delegate from Mississippi, was seated at a table next to ours. Fred asked if we had heard about a jet flying into the World Trade Center earlier that morning. Neither of us had, but I remember saying that I had read about planes crashing into the Empire State Building in years past. I had not only been in this skyscraper during a visit to the 1964 World's Fair but had also recently been atop one of the Trade Center towers.

A few minutes after hearing the news, a restaurant waiter told us that a second plane had flown into the Trade Center. Moments later the Pentagon, less than three miles away, exploded into flame and rubble. Although we could neither see nor hear this tragedy unfold, all of us were wondering where the next strike would be.

As discovery of al Qaeda's intended targets later revealed, I was closer to death than I had even imagined. The terrorists' final bombing site was the Capitol Building—ten blocks away! But for the heroic passengers of UAL Flight 93, who overpowered the terrorists, crashed the plane into a field near Shanksville, Pennsylvania, and sacrificed their lives, I am now certain I would have died on September 11. I cannot express how I feel. It is too hard and painful to contemplate.

Despite the ensuing fear and confusion, the delegates convened later in the morning for introductions and preparation. Kevin Brennan was the foundation coordinator for the meeting. He asked each of us to write a one-page paper summarizing our experience with inflammatory arthritis, the treatments we had tried, and our need for access to better therapies such as Enbrel. We had come from Arizona, Colorado, Connecticut, Mississippi, Vermont, Montana, Arkansas, Florida, California, New Jersey, West Virginia, Utah, Texas, Washington, Alaska, and most significant, New York City and Washington, D.C. Regrettably, our stories were never shared with our Members of Congress the next day, September 12.

It didn't take long before the harsh reality of that terrible day led to the cancellation of what had been a most promising event. Getting home from D.C. proved problematic for almost all the delegates, and I was no exception. All flights everywhere were cancelled. It took a week before I could finally get home. On the bright side, however, both Monica and Matt were in the East, she working for Americorps in Baltimore and he doing his junior year exchange at the University of Massachusetts in Amherst. Monica and I drove her car to Amherst where we tried to decompress from the living nightmare. There was a rugby tournament involving several New England universities and colleges, one of which was the University of Maine. As a way of meeting other students during her junior year exchange there, Monica turned out for rugby, a game she had never played before. By the weekend following September 11, she had been away from this brutal sport for two years. Nonetheless, her former Maine teammates cajoled her into playing for them. With no helmet and only a teeth protector, shin guards, and cleats, Monica joined her teammates on the field of play. Even though I had never witnessed my beautiful daughter playing such a violent game, seeing her run down and tackle her opponents so easily reaffirmed my unbiased conviction that she is an accomplished athlete. Watching her play was a welcome respite from the rigors of that time, and even though she had been battered and bruised from play, she said at our evening meal, "I hurt, Dad, but it's a good hurt."

Monica played soccer and softball. She was fun to watch, especially on corner kicks. I personally witnessed my dear daughter banana kick the ball from the corner box past the outstretched body of the hapless goalie and into the net. My brother said of her softball prowess, "She could hit the snot out of the ball and run down any fly in the outfield capable of being caught."

Matt is no slouch either. He has successfully ascended Mount Rainier, the 14,410-foot jewel-in-the-crown peak of the rugged, magnificent Cascade Mountain Range, on his first and second climbs. He has scuba dived at night with manta rays, the gentle, giant denizens of the deep, off the coast of Maui. Most of all, I am proudest to be his old timer as a result of his participation in the foundation's Great

West Region Inaugural People's Coast Classic. Starting in Astoria and ending in Brookings, it is a scenic 363-mile fundraising bicycle tour along the incomparable Oregon Coast, but the coast road can be extremely dangerous in windy, wet weather, and my heart was in my throat during the last leg from Port Orford to Brookings. Matt's bike broke down and he was soaking wet, but once it was repaired, he bicycled on. Yes, he has my stubborn Irish gene, in spades!

As the all-too-brief weekend came to a close, Monica and I shared our final meal with Matt and then departed for Baltimore. At last I had made my return flight bookings to Spokane. After arriving at the Baltimore-Washington airport, all of us passengers suffered the agonizing indignity of "enhanced security measures" before we were allowed to proceed to the departure gates. The scale of confiscation of the personal property of American airline passengers was unprecedented at that time. Even my nail clippers were seized. For the very first time, I looked suspiciously at all the other passengers, during both legs of my flight to Spokane, fearful that any one of them might commandeer the aircraft and crash it into a building. It was a long flight home. I had been rerouted, though, from Los Angeles to Chicago. Just as my presence on the East Coast has been a blessing for my family and me on what will forever be remembered as 9/11, it is also a blessing for me personally that my flight home had stopped in Chicago. I will never forget the refuge my beloved cousin, Babs, provided me there.

Babs and I have been close ever since we knew the other existed. Her mother, Ramona, was my father's sister. During World War II, Aunt Ramona and Babs's brother, Bruce, lived with my mother and brother for the duration of the war. Uncle John and my father had volunteered, and their duties took them to far-flung duty stations. Babs and I weren't even a glint in our fathers' eyes during their voluntary but hard separation from our mothers and brothers. We are "baby boomers," members of the generation our parents spawned in record-shattering numbers immediately after the war.

Along with my other cousins, Bruce, Susan, and Mary, Babs grew up in Richmond, Indiana. Even though "it's more than 2,000 miles all the way" from Spokane, our families stayed constantly in touch with one another. We spent alternating summer vacations fastening the family ties even tighter. As a result, Babs is my closest cousin.

As I write this chapter of my memoir, the haunting lyrics of *Gimme Shelter* play over in my mind. The apocalyptic verses, which the Stones memorialized in their classic recording decades before, express so succinctly how I felt on September 11, 2001. I was at the epicenter of that date's horrors and I honestly believed then that I might not survive. The "threat'ning storm" broke over the entire country that fateful day. Consequently, the legislation proposed by Senator Murray and Congresswoman Dunn to improve the lives of several million Americans with arthritis did eventually "fade away."

Notwithstanding the portent of 9/11, Monica sounded an optimistic note. Two months after the tragedies of that terrible day, she decided upon a career in pharmacy. As part of her application process to various schools, she said the most important factor in her decision to become a pharmacist was what she personally saw from the benefits of my Enbrel therapy. Based on the early results of my taking Enbrel, she said it had made a huge difference in my life and the lives of our family, and, most important, had dramatically improved the quality of my life. What better testimonial is there than my loving daughter's? She therefore wants to be involved in the treatment and cure for rheumatoid arthritis. She then concluded her application saying, "Pharmacy would allow me the opportunity not only to make a difference in the life of my father but also in the lives of people in my community."

Monica was admitted to the University of Maryland School of Pharmacy in August 2002. As part of her course requirement in human biology, she reviewed the very same medical journal article I had discussed with Dr. Stevenson nearly four years earlier. Published in the *Annals of Internal Medicine* and entitled "Etanercept Therapy in Rheumatoid Arthritis: A Randomized, Controlled Trial" co-authored by Dr. Scott Baumgartner, it detailed the results of the Enbrel drug trials conducted in Spokane and elsewhere across the country. The article prompted my daughter to speak with me about my experiences with Enbrel and the improvements this drug enabled me to make. In 2006 Monica graduated *cum laude* and is now a hospital pharmacist.

Chapter 21

Becoming a Public Advocate

Humor has helped me in many different ways.
It is the most serious form of seeking and maintaining perspective.
—Sol Levy, M.D.

Vivian's father gave his advice to members of the Washington State Bar Association during their annual convention in September 1978. A forensic psychiatrist practicing in Spokane, his last public address, entitled "Law & Psychiatry," concerned mental-capacity defenses and the psychiatrist's role as an expert witness in a criminal trial. Suffering from the painful cancer that would claim his life two months later, he nonetheless wove the importance of humor throughout his remarks to illustrate its usefulness in his work. Having learned that humor relaxes tension and steers midway between gravity and levity, he told the audience he was the prototypical psychiatrist: a Jewish doctor who couldn't stand the sight of blood!

My father-in-law's counsel reinforced my own sense of humor. Bred into me by my Irish ancestry, I've found it an absolute necessity in dealing with my JRA. My children too have learned the importance of it. Monica has given me the complete DVD series of John Mortimer's wonderful *Rumpole of the Bailey* stories. Played superbly by Leo McKern, Horace Rumpole, a "junior British barrister with forty years of life at the bar," relishes the cynical skewering of judges, chambers colleagues, and police officers. He is also constantly thwarting his wife, Hilda, whom he calls, under his breath, "she who must be obeyed," in her relentless schemes of trying to elevate him from his lowly status as "an Old Bailey hack" to the lofty heights of "high court red judge." My sympathetic daughter has also given me the complete DVD series of *Black Adder,* the British historical sitcom featuring the satirical wit of Rowan Atkinson; and Matt has given me *The Complete Far Side,* the wonderfully bound two-volume treasure of Gary Larson's pithy cartoons. Many a time the thoughtfulness of my children's gifts has helped smooth out the rough edges of my bad days.

I called upon humor to illustrate the importance of carrying on after 9/11. Just as Vivian's father had employed humor in his address to the Washington State Bar Association on its importance in life, I also used it when the Arthritis Foundation convened its 2002 Advocacy Summit. In the program segment, "Becoming an Effective Advocate," I portrayed the fictional Senator Grumpy from Pennsylvania. The director of clinical research for the University of Pittsburgh Arthritis Institute played my constituent. Her role was to overcome my curmudgeonly resistance to supporting increased appropriations for arthritis research at a time when defense spending and homeland security consumed a major portion of our national treasure. For the most part, I followed the script. Even when I deviated from it and threw the good doctor a curveball, she hit it out of the park. We enjoyed ourselves, and the laughter from the audience showed their appreciation of comic relief during this grave period in our nation's history.

At the 2003 Advocacy Summit, I was one of four speakers on the topic of "Living Well with Rheumatoid Arthritis." My fellow panelists were all physicians, specializing in rheumatology, orthopedic surgery, and rehabilitation. My perspective was that of a patient advocate. I again used humor to illustrate its absolute necessity, especially in times of adversity, which rheumatoid arthritis patients must have in dealing with their condition. I relied upon the tale of "The Football Game Between The Big Animals and The Little Animals" to make my case.

One day the Big Animals challenged the Little Animals to a football game. The Big Animals won the coin toss, kicked off, and the drubbing of the Little Animals was on. By the end of the first half, the score was Big Animals 49, Little Animals 0.

During the half-time locker room break, the exasperated coach of the Little Animals pleaded with his despondent players to at least try to stop the Big Animals from getting a first down in the second half, but everyone except Centipede the Linebacker, formerly with the Baltimore Colts, believed this was impossible. With the sole exception of Centipede, the Little Animals and their coach walked dejectedly back to the field and kicked off for the second half.

For the very first time in the game, the Little Animals kept the Big Animals from returning the ball for yet another touchdown. Not only that, but on the first play from scrimmage, Rhinoceros the Running Back was stopped for no gain. Determined to score on the next play, Hippo the Quarterback arrogantly called for keeping the ball after the snap. Not only was he dropped dead in his tracks, but to his great chagrin, he was also tackled behind the line of scrimmage. The coach of the Big Animals was so disgusted with this change in momentum he immediately called for a time out to mercilessly harangue his players and send in the next play. It was a complete waste of time. On a double reverse, Elephant the End was not only shamefully tackled ten yards behind the line of scrimmage but also fumbled the ball. The Little Animals pounced on it at the five-yard line. At this strange turn of events, the perplexed coach of the Little Animals called a time out. After his players gathered around, the coach asked, "Who stopped Rhinoceros?"

Confidently, Centipede answered, "I did, Coach."

"Who tackled Hippo?" the coach asked.

Centipede exclaimed, "I did, Coach!"

Incredulous at Centipede's success, the coach nevertheless asked, "Then who brought down Elephant?"

Emphatically, Centipede yelled, "I did, Coach!"

"Then where were you in the first half?" the coach exploded angrily.

To which Centipede nonchalantly replied, "I was in the locker room lacing up my cleats."

Like Centipede, rheumatoid arthritis patients, given the right treatment, can be very effective. It just takes a little longer to get going in the daily game of life.

Chapter 22

Perseverance Through Adversity

To strive, to seek, to find, and not to yield.
—Alfred Tennyson

Shortly after I returned home from the 2003 Arthritis Foundation Advocacy Summit, two memorable events occurred within days of one another: the death of Vivian's mother and the start of the second war in Iraq.

Erika Levy, affectionately known in her later years as "Grandma," lived a long and interesting life. Born to wealthy parents in 1914, she enjoyed the advantages such status conferred, but soon after their wedding in 1938, she and Sol would flee Nazi Germany and start over in America. Here they would raise their children in a far safer country and do what all good parents do: Prepare them for the good times and the bad through unconditional love and experiential wisdom. Widowed at age sixty-four, she continued to enjoy life greatly, especially in the company of her grandchildren. Whether vacationing with them in far-flung places or conjuring up Swiss chocolate—anywhere and anytime—for their "sweet tooth," she showered on them the affection and attention only a doting grandma could. From a life of joy and leisure to, in the blink of an eye, a life of sadness and toil, she came full-circle during her eighty-eight years. After a brief illness, she died, as she was fond of saying, with "all her marbles."

As for the start of the second war in Iraq, it was, in the inimitable words of Yogi Berra, *"déjà vu* all over again." The war in Afghanistan made the work of arthritis advocates daunting to say the least.

Evidence of this was the failure to pass the bill reintroduced by Senator Murray during the 108th Congress for Medicare coverage of self-injected biologics. The remark I made during the delivery of my address to colleagues three weeks before the bombing of Baghdad proved regrettably true:

> With the threat of war looming and a record-setting federal deficit facing the nation in the next fiscal year, it looks difficult, does it not, for us to convince Congress to act in our best interests. And being unpaid advocates matched against well-heeled lobbyists, the challenge to secure federal funds for our causes seems insurmountable.

On the eve of the debate in the Senate regarding the resolution to invade Iraq, I sent an email to Senator Murray urging her to vote against it. Not knowing then that the stated reason for going to war, i.e., weapons of mass destruction, was meritless, I nevertheless said there would be more economic hardship for ordinary Americans should the United States attack Iraq. Despite Senator Murray's opposition to the resolution, the Senate passed it—and the war came.

The country was still going through the economic fallout of the 2000 dot-com collapse. With ramped-up spending on homeland security and the Afghanistan war coming on the heels of the technology-stock bubble bust, another war on a much larger scale would set back even further the accomplishment of the foundation's legislative agenda. To their credit the foundation was able to secure changes in Medicare by creating an opportunity for rheumatoid and psoriatic arthritis patients to get coverage for expensive biologic therapies such as Enbrel, but enrollment in the demonstration program was limited to a small number of patients with these conditions. Thus the program did not cover all eligible Americans, which the legislative proposals of Senator Murray and Congresswoman Dunn to expand Medicare would have.

The disappointment I experienced during my initial foray into the world of public health policy did not deter me. I soldiered on for the foundation and occasionally called to mind the U.S. Postal Service motto I paraphrased while speaking at the 2003 Advocacy

Summit: *Neither rain, nor sleet, nor budget woes would keep me from my appointed rounds.* But as the new millennium's first years unfolded, other commitments took center stage for a time. While my health waxed, my parents', into their eighties, waned. The dread of their deaths increasingly pressed upon me, and once they suffered fractures from falls in their home, my role in their care increased substantially. Fortunately, I was winding down my law practice and therefore could devote more time and energy to their needs.

Having endured the financial stresses of the Great Depression and the rationing of World War II in their young lives, my parents nevertheless reaped the benefits of the financial prudence they had developed during their productive years. Consequently, they were able to live out their lives comfortably in the home they had built in 1950. After a brief hospital stay, my father died at age eighty-seven. My mother followed him two years later, at eighty-eight, in her own home. This was what she wanted.

It's hard to be objective about one's own parents. Evidence of this observation is readily available in the obituary columns. Nonetheless, I hope the brief account I give of my parents is as free from bias as I can make it.

James Henry Lynch:
January 21, 1918–August 22, 2005

My loving father was born in Spokane. He did many things in his life, but I believe the best thing he ever did was wed my dear mother. Though their upbringing was different in many ways, their love for one another overcame the obstacles they encountered during their sixty-four years as husband and wife.

Four children were born to my parents. The death of my older sister, Betty Ann, at the age of four months, was a particularly painful loss for my mother, coming as it did in 1942 when my father was in the U.S. Army Air Corps. Though he never spoke to me about Betty Ann, I know her death affected him. I am very fortunate to have been spared the deep sadness my parents suffered the rest of their lives.

My father's childhood was marred by the sadness of another death. When he was six years old, his father, James Henry Lynch, died from a heart attack at age seventy. With his mother, Anna Fitzpatrick Lynch, then forty, and his younger sisters, four-year-old Ramona, and two-year-old Margie, living in their home on West 24th Avenue in Spokane, the challenges for my father growing up without his father must have been very acute — but he met them. More lay ahead when his mother died, at age fifty-four, while my father was at the University of Notre Dame. Yet he again rose to the occasion: He saw that his sisters did not lack the guidance their mother had provided. He protected them during their minority and carefully managed his mother's estate until they came of age.

Although the Great Depression did not visit upon my father the economic hardships so many others suffered, the loss of his father quickly brought home the responsibilities of being frugal. Thus my father was schooled at an early age to be thrifty. The lessons he learned paid off. My mother was more secure for this virtue of my father.

Still, no one is perfect. My father made his living on the road. He was a good provider, but spending time together with a parent, especially when young, is more precious than gold. Although we would fish together on opening day and travel to many places during family vacations, I would have liked very much to have gotten to know him better at dinnertime. I am certain I would have learned a lot, not just about him but also about life, yet I do not begrudge my father these lost opportunities. In a way, his absences aided me in developing my independent point of view. By standing back, he allowed me to be my own pathfinder. The philosophical compass I have used has not always been true, but my journey with it has been interesting and rewarding.

When Vivian and I announced our intention to marry, my father, a devout Irish Catholic, could have objected. Vivian is Jewish, and the Catholic Church then taught that the sacrament of matrimony could not be conferred upon our marriage. Despite this prohibition for practicing Catholics, my father did not object. In fact, he supported me.

My father possessed many of the virtues Lincoln possessed, but the one for which I am most grateful was his not questioning an important decision once I had made it. Yes, as a father, he corrected me in my youth when called for; he would have failed me had he not; but by letting me exercise my judgment, he helped me become a man.

⸻ ◦◦◦ ⸻

Margaret Olive Shannon Lynch: February 2, 1919–November 2, 2007

My loving mother was born Ground Hog's Day in Chapeau, Quebec. The fourth of nine children, she and her six surviving siblings grew up in Pembroke, Ontario, just on the other side of the Ottawa River from Chapeau. Unlike my father's childhood, my mother's was filled with economic hardship. Because her father could neither read nor write, steady employment, especially during the Great Depression, was problematic. The consequences for my mother were at times severe, but they forged in her a determination to have a better life. She thus became a registered nurse in 1940. My mother was the primary caregiver in our family. With my father away on his work in Idaho and Montana, occasionally up to three weeks at a time, my mother raised my siblings and me alone. It was tough duty for her at times, but we not only survived but also thrived, and as we passed from childhood through adolescence to adulthood, she kept the home beacon glowing.

Despite having to discipline us far more often than our father did, my mother was fun to be with. Some of the stories in *Growing Up Rich*, the autobiography of her youth, ghostwritten by my father, showed just how much of a daredevil and thrill seeker she was — whether it was jumping barefooted on and off a moving train; running on an Ottawa River log boom and surviving a fall from it; or saving her old horse, Dan, after he fell through the river's ice while pulling her in a sleigh. Even at age forty-three, she learned how to water-ski and continued to slalom, inside the wake, until she was sixty.

At my mother's funeral service in St. Augustine's Church, where my father, brother, sister, and I were baptized, made our first confession, received our first communion, and finally were confirmed by the bishop of the Spokane diocese, I spoke on behalf of our family. At the conclusion of my remembrances, I compared my mother to three Biblical heroines: Ruth, a devoted mother and the great grandmother of David; Esther, the noble Queen of Persia; and Deborah, a great *shaphat* (judge) of Israel. All were loving and beautiful women, and they possessed many virtues, especially fidelity, courage, and wisdom, but what I learned most from reading their stories to my mother during her final year, and from the lessons she taught me during my formative years, is the virtue of perseverance through adversity.

My mother's nursing duties at Shriners Hospital were the most influential experiences for me; from them sprang the gift of learning the virtue of perseverance through adversity. I am most grateful to my mother for bestowing it upon me. It was she who taught me, through word and deed, just how important it would be in dealing with my JRA.

Even though my parents' needs took more of my time during the last years of their lives, I continued my advocacy duties for the foundation. From 2001 to 2011, I attended every Advocacy Summit in Washington, D.C. My role was essentially the same each year: Learn about the foundation's legislative agenda and pitch it to members of Congress. Unlike the rookie advocates, I didn't have to tell my personal story. My congressional representatives already knew it. I would invariably follow up with them by letter after I returned home from each summit. Occasionally I, along with other local advocates, particularly mothers and their children with JA, visited Representative Cathy McMorris Rodgers when she was in our district. From 2004 to 2010 the main topic for discussion was the bipartisan bill, introduced in both the Senate and the House of Representatives as the Arthritis Prevention, Control, and Cure Act.

The statistics supporting passage of the Act are staggering. With more than a hundred different forms of the disease, nearly one in every three American adults of every age suffers from arthritis or chronic joint problems. 300,000 children also live with the pain, disability, and emotional trauma caused by JA. With so many Americans affected by the leading cause of disability, the annual cost of arthritis, in medical expenses, lost earnings, and reduced productivity is $156 billion. Early diagnosis, treatment, and appropriate management of this chronic condition are critical in controlling symptoms and improving quality of life. The Arthritis Prevention, Control, and Cure Act represented the most significant federal effort to address arthritis in a generation. It called for:

♦ Enhancing the National Arthritis Action Plan by providing additional support to federal, state, and private efforts to prevent and manage arthritis;

♦ Developing a National Arthritis Education and Outreach Campaign to educate the healthcare profession on successful self-management strategies for controlling arthritis;

♦ Ensuring greater coordination and intensification of federal research efforts by organizing a National Arthritis and Rheumatic Diseases Summit;

♦ Providing greater attention to the area of JA research through the creation of planning grants for innovative research specific to JA; and

♦ Creating incentives to encourage health professionals to enter the field of pediatric rheumatology through the establishment of an education loan repayment and career development award program.

To say the least, the breadth and depth of this legislative proposal dwarfed the thirty-word amendment proposed by Senator Murray and Congresswoman Dunn for the expansion of Medicare coverage to self-injected biologics. It was the most ambitious effort by the foundation and was supported by many professional healthcare provider associations, hospitals, and other foundations. The act held great promise for me and for millions of other Americans, so, during the next seven years, I put my oar in and rowed strenuously for passage.

Groundswell for making the act law increased among members of Congress. Cosponsors were added in each new session. With their small army of volunteer advocates and the support of the public, the efforts of the foundation looked like they would pay off. By the end of 2010, the act had finally passed in the House of Representatives. Representative Rodgers voted for it. Just after the mid-term elections, I wrote to Senator Murray, a senior member of the Senate committee considering the act, and urged the exercise of her authority "to mark up the bill for enactment by the Senate." On November 29, 2010, her aide called me and said that since the bill was not on the agenda of the executive committee, the Arthritis Prevention, Control, and Cure Act would not pass. I was crestfallen.

Chapter 23

Success From Failure

Never, ever give up.
—Diana Nyad

On September 2, 2013, at the age of sixty-four, Diana Nyad finally completed a 110-mile swim from Havana, Cuba, to Key West, Florida. Her four previous attempts, beginning in 1978, to cover this vast expanse of the Caribbean Sea had failed. Absent from this successful open-water crossing were the poisonous jellyfish stings, asthma attacks, and bad weather which had plagued this long-distance veteran's earlier attempts. Dazed, wobbly, sunburned, and disoriented, her message on emerging from the sea serves as an inspiration to everyone on how to achieve success despite prior failures. Because of her courageous crossing in the treacherous Caribbean waters, she motivated me to participate in the much smaller, and certainly less hazardous, 1.4-mile Lake Washington Park-to-Park Crossing, in August 2014, as well as the 2015 Lake Coeur d'Alene Triathlon and the 2015 Lake Coeur d'Alene Crossing. The Crossing, set at 2.4 miles—the distance Iron Men and Women competitors swim—was anything but 2.4 miles because the course markers meandered. Wind, waves, and intersecting lake channels extended the distance to at least three miles, but I survived and crossed the finish line—at age sixty-eight.

Even though my earnest efforts and those of many others had failed to produce passage of the Arthritis Prevention, Control, and Cure Act, I did not give up volunteer activities to try to make a difference in the lives of Americans with arthritis, especially those of Katfish. To be sure there were several factors that no amount of advocacy could overcome: wars abroad, security at home, and the global Great Recession. Even before Senator Murray's aide had delivered the dispiriting news, the sledding had been rough, and in light of the act's demise, the foundation scaled down their legislative agenda, but as Nyad's story exemplifies, success can come from failure.

For my part I was in relatively good health during the first decade of the new millennium. Enbrel and then Simponi, a similar drug, stopped the downward spiral, and with the shutdown of my law practice in 2009 and the closure of my mother's estate in 2010, I knew I could do more about improving my own life and the lives of all Katfish.

To improve my own life, I set upon a course I had last navigated in 1988. At the age of sixty-two, I wanted to see if I could once again swim 1.5 km in an open water competition, but just as it was then, I needed help. It would take a team effort to accomplish my goal. I turned to my children who willingly agreed to be my teammates, Matt as the 40 km cyclist and Monica as the 10 km runner, in the 2010 Lake Coeur d'Alene Triathlon. They chose to call us the Snail Darters 2, in honor of my first team, the Snail Darters.

It was my brother's idea to register our 1985 team as the Snail Darters. A tiny fish discovered in the Little Tennessee River, the snail darter's habitat was about to be destroyed by construction of a dam. In 1978, however, the U.S. Supreme Court ruled that the fish was protected by the Endangered Species Act, thereby preventing for a while the damming of the river. The lengthy and costly struggle to save this scavenger of snails means many things to many people involved with environmental matters, and its name has even been adopted to describe the war over water usage as "snail darter politics," but for me the fish symbolized the plight of all Katfish who, until recently, have relied upon adults for the prevention, control, and cure of juvenile arthritis.

From 2010 to 2013, my children and I completed four triathlons as the Snail Darters 2. Matt and I also participated in two aquathlons, I as the swimmer and he as the cyclist, under the team name, Snail Darters 2-1, in recognition that we were missing Monica. Both of these competitions were held at the Grand Columbian Triathlon at

Coulee Dam on the Columbia River. I consider myself very fortunate to have been able to participate in these events with Monica and Matt, especially because I couldn't do much athletically with them in their earlier years. I hope they have come to see me as Jem and Scout saw their father, Atticus, after the mad dog encounter in Harper Lee's classic novel *To Kill A Mockingbird*—old maybe, but not so feeble.

As for improvement in the lives of Katfish, my interest in their plight began long before I ramped up my service for the foundation in 2010. On Valentine's Day 2002, I read an article in the local news-paper about Kelly Norris, a high school gymnast who has JRA. Her story reminded me of the difficulties I had at her age.

By contacting Kelly through her coach, I was able to learn what she was doing to deal with the daily struggles of JRA. She was on the waiting list for Enbrel, so she was still suffering through the trials of the standard drug regimen. While the article shined a light on JRA, what struck me as sad was her comment to me that she didn't have anyone to talk to who understood her situation. The foundation set out to do something about this problem for Kelly and other Katfish.

Starting in 2004 the foundation believed that the health and well-being of kids and teens with JA necessitated including not only parents but also siblings in a support program. What the foundation learned over the years is that giving kids and teens a chance to meet other children with similar conditions helps them (and their families) become more resilient. Furthermore, the foundation also discovered that Katfish summer camps are a treasure for their volunteers who did not have a chance to make these connections in the old days.

A natural outcome of the Katfish program was the inclusion of Katfish and their families at the Advocacy Summits, beginning in 2004. The hope was that the telling of their stories to members of Con-gress would be the beginning of a lifelong commitment to advocacy. As I had expressed to Kelly, there won't be a cure for her and other Katfish unless they focus the nation's attention and resources upon JA. The Kids' Summits were designed to do just that, and so it was that I began learning about Katfish and their families. I had finally found my tribe, even though it was far into my adult years—better late than never!

At the 2005 Advocacy Summit I met Taylor Bruce and her parents, Courtney and Mike, from Tacoma, Washington. Taylor, who loves rescuing dogs and cats, had been hit hard with JRA when she was just eighteen months old. I told her story in *InHealthNW* (July–August, 2006), a Spokane health magazine.

Although Taylor had begun to walk, JRA forced her to revert to crawling. Her pediatrician put her in the hospital where she suffered through IV antibiotic therapy, a bone scan, joint taps, and blood draws. Two months later, a pediatric rheumatologist finally diagnosed her condition. Even with intensive treatment, JRA affects her hands, knees, ankles, and jaw. One treatment drug, cortisone, eroded the joint in her right jaw for which she underwent surgery during adolescence.

In 2011 I met the Gonzales family from Moses Lake, Washington. Riley, a typical boy who loves helicopters and airplanes, suffers from the same fate as Taylor. I told his story in *InHealthNW* (November–December, 2011).

Riley was born with JRA; his condition went undetected after his left ankle swelled from an accidental fall when he was just eleven months old. Acting on his pediatrician's advice, Riley's parents, Brooke and James, rushed him from their Moses Lake home to Spokane, a distance of more than a hundred miles. Further examination and MRI testing led to one option—surgery.

Following the operation and two-week hospitalization, a peripherally inserted central catheter (PICC) line was put into Riley for a possible bone infection. This invasive procedure, in which a catheter is inserted through the veins until the tip rests in the heart, was complicated by his little arms and small veins. The first attempted insertion swelled his right arm and the second attempt caused a blood clot. It was only after the third insertion into his left arm that the procedure was successful.

During the four months of excruciating PICC therapy, Riley's doctors ultimately diagnosed his JRA. Following this course of treatment, his testing and procedures included bone scans, MRIs, steroid IVs, cortisone injections, and oral prescription medicines. This extensive therapy has helped control his JRA, but Riley's parents, as indeed other parents just like them, are legitimately concerned that their other children will be diagnosed with JRA.

I came to learn more about Katfish and their families during the foundation's annual Arthritis Walks and Katfish Camps. The latter events bring children together, from toddlers to teens, to engage in a wide range of activities, the most important of which is making new friends who truly understand what living with arthritis means. Campers also take part in activities to help them increase self-confidence, improve arthritis self-management, and develop leadership skills. As a speaker at one of the camps, I urged the Katfish and their families to do what I had advised Kelly to do: Through the power of their collective Katfish voices, focus the nation's attention and resources on JA so that a cure would be found.

Starting in 2010, the importance of the foundation's advocacy work took on new meaning for me. Even though I believe the cure will not be discovered in my lifetime, I am determined to make it so during the lives of the current Katfish. I became a member of the foundation's Pacific Northwest Chapter Board of Directors and the patient advocate on their National Research Strategy Committee's Juvenile Arthritis Task Force. Both were three-year commitments, with duties ranging from advocacy to fundraising. Even though my terms expired at the end of 2012, I continue my volunteer activities with the foundation's Spokane Jingle Bell Run & Walk Committee.

Chapter 24

Profiles in Courage

Courage: The state or quality of mind or spirit that enables one to face danger, fear, or vicissitudes with self-possession, confidence, and resolution.
—The American Heritage Dictionary

The Story of Christina McCarty

I met Christina and her parents, Jeanne and Dennis, at the Arthritis Foundation's 2006 Katfish Camp near Auburn, Washington. I was a guest speaker on the role of advocacy for Katfish and their families. Our introduction began at mealtime. It was then that I learned about Christina's juvenile arthritis and that the McCarty family hailed from Spokane. Little did I know then what a roller coaster ride the McCarty family had been on and what they were in for.

I first learned about Christina at the foundation's 2005 Spokane Arthritis Walk in May. She was the honoree and I was manning the Advocacy Booth. She wasn't the first Katfish I had met, but she was among the first of the tribe I was about to join. I didn't, however, see this pivotal encounter coming then.

Jeanne and Dennis had been involved with the foundation as organizers in the first series of the Spokane Jingle Bell Run & Walk fundraisers. By the time I began my volunteer duties, this event had ended, but not so for my association with the McCarty family. In fact, Jeanne and I were instrumental in bringing the Run & Walk back. The irony was that neither of us knew about this twist of fate in 2006. That's the beauty of kismet—it was meant to happen.

Since our first meeting, the McCarty family has shown me just how important it is to bring awareness not only to Christina's JA but to the JA of all Katfish. The McCarty family is deeply committed and passionate about making this happen so that the cure will be found for JA in Christina's lifetime. I want this as well for Christina and all the other Katfish.

In 2010 I joined the Spokane JBRW Committee where I got the low down on just how great the committee is in making the Spokane community not only aware of the pervasiveness of arthritis, especially in children, but also in raising funds for the prevention, control, and cure of this insidious and lifelong disease. But when my tour of duty ended in 2013, I decided to resign from the committee and concentrate on my own mission: raising awareness about JA and helping to find the cure. Then I learned in August 2014 just how ill Christina had become because of her JA. I was shocked! At the first opportunity Vivian and I visited Christina at St. Luke's Rehabilitation Institute. She was an inpatient there because she could not be discharged to her home following a lengthy in-patient stay at Sacred Heart Medical Center. A life-threatening disease had invaded her body and had changed her so completely that we couldn't believe the transformation. Her voice was unrecognizable and she needed a wheelchair to get around. I then determined that I would return to the committee and resume what I do best: advocate, advocate, advocate!

Christina is a fourteen-year-old 8th grader whose artwork of the Old Katfish graces the cover of this memoir. Here is her story:

—————

My parents tell me I crawled, walked, talked, and giggled just like every other healthy kid. In 2003, when I was eighteen months old, I went to the hospital because of an infection. It started like a normal cold, but because it got worse, I was taken to the emergency room. When I got there, I had another ear infection. It was mastoiditis. After I started on amoxicillin for this, I had an allergic reaction to this medicine, so my hospital stay lasted five days, which was five days too long! After I was discharged from the hospital, I had to get stronger in order to have another set of ear tubes put in and my adenoids removed.

After the 2003 hospital visit, my mom and dad started noticing something different about me. When I walked, I dragged one of my legs. My knees were noticeably swollen, my fingers hard to bend, and I had tears. My parents talked with our doctor, and, after a year of seeing other doctors and going through the process of elimination, the diagnosis of JRA was made.

On April 26, 2005, my journey into the long adventure of the autoimmune world began. My parents and I were so lucky to meet Dr. Meredith Heick, a rheumatologist, to start my treatment. Her schedule was so full, though, that she met with us after hours. This first visit started me on the routine of methotrexate tablets and 24/7 children's Motrin. I also had knee injections at Shriners Hospital to bring down the inflammation. I also started occupational, physical, and pool therapy at St. Luke's Rehabilitation Institute as an outpatient. I was three and a half years old.

Mornings started with pain and stiffness in my joints. I usually took a warm bath to ease the pain. Breakfast was always in bed or in the bathtub. My mom was able to change her work hours so I could get a warm bath, do water stretching, and soak before heading off to daycare. We also discovered the Salvation Army's therapy pool. At that time it was the only warm-water pool open to the public. I spent Saturday mornings there.

Just as we were leaving Dr. Heick's office one day in May 2005, Mom picked up a flyer for an upcoming Arthritis Walk in Spokane. We marked the date in our calendar. This was the beginning of our new "team." I chose the name "Christina's Butterflies." We rallied family and friends to join us that day. We met Johanna Lindsay from the Arthritis Foundation's office in Seattle. She in turn introduced us to the foundation, the American Juvenile Arthritis Organization, and the KAT-Camp. The AJAO's annual conference was at Providence, Rhode Island, in July, so we went to it because the foundation sponsored us.

The conference was incredible and exhausting as this world of arthritis was still new to us.

In August 2006 we went to the foundation's KAT-Camp. KAT-Camp is held every summer in the Seattle area. Our first camp was amazing. I was able to meet other kids with arthritis, and my parents met other parents who were dealing with the same problems as mine. In addition to learning about JA, all of the Katfish had so many fun activities and a talent show. Our first camp was also memorable because we met John Lynch. John's compassion, knowledge, and leadership in advocacy have been incredible for our family.

As my first year with JA went by, I was still on Motrin and methotrexate. If Mom could get this drug into me, my swelling and pain weren't so bad. She'd also crush the awful tasting methotrexate and try to disguise it in my food. Most of the time she couldn't get me to take it this way, and then I started on methotrexate shots. They were terrible. I threw up after every shot because they made me sick. Sundays were my shot days and Monday mornings were my worst days.

After my first year in the world of rheumatology ended, Mom again signed us up for the 2006 Arthritis Walk in Spokane. I was the honoree. This was my first time to be an honoree. Our family, friends, Dr. Heick, and John Lynch rallied around us with tons of support.

In 2007 I started having more ear infections. Also, one of my eardrums ruptured, and I had to have my third pair of ear tubes put in. Every time I got an infection, I needed more antibiotics, but I didn't have to get the methotrexate shots, because they weakened my immune system. Once the antibiotics worked, I got the shots again. I was on another roller coaster ride!

In 2009 I had to get Enbrel shots every week along with my methotrexate shots and Motrin. I still threw up and I was tired every Monday morning because of the nausea. Anyway, I also started warm soaks and stretching. I learned how to adapt my body to do what I wanted to do, but sometimes no matter what I tried, I couldn't adapt because of my JA. My elbows hurt so much they wouldn't straighten out. They would freeze up and I would lose range of motion. Then Shriners stopped their clinic. My JA went from bad to worse. It was terrible for me!

In 2010 my inflammation was under control. I was able to stop methotrexate and just be on Enbrel. By the end of 2013 I was in total remission and was able to stop Enbrel, too. No more shots! I had a great six months, but in May 2014 I hurt my ankle. It swelled up, and on top of that I got a swollen knee, so I started Enbrel again.

In August I told Mom my feet hurt and I couldn't dance. I love to dance, but my JA was so bad I didn't have the strength to do it. My eyes were also bothering me. My pediatrician said my eye exam was good, but my blood pressure was elevated. I got lethargic right after the visit, and my vision got worse. About two weeks later my eyesight was really bad, so I had a blood test. It showed I had mononucleosis, and my left eye drooped. No wonder I felt the way I did! Next stop was the Sacred Heart Medical Center ER. My blood pressure was sky high. Mom asked the nurse if the reading was right. It was and the doctor immediately came to my bed. I was so scared!

I was put in the pediatric ICU. I didn't have a stroke or brain tumor, but I did have the Epstein-Barr virus, which caused the mononucleosis and Bell's palsy. This is why I was so lethargic and had the drooping on the left side of my face. The drooping got so bad that my left eye and the left side of my mouth wouldn't close. The virus also attacked my peripheral nervous system. My blood pressure and heart rate were very high, and I lost weight, so IVs were put into my arms for my high blood pressure and pain.

Eventually I got out of the ICU and was put on the pediatric floor, but the lethargy, pain, eye problems, and weight loss continued. When I was finally released to St. Luke's, I had been at Sacred Heart for ten days, but I couldn't walk, so I was put in a wheelchair and taken by transport. But I still had to have the IVs at St. Luke's and needed a wheelchair to go to physical therapy, occupational therapy, recreational therapy, and speech therapy. This was so hard because I had zero energy.

The big challenge for me at St. Luke's was to try and hold on to what muscle I had and to not end up on a feeding tube, and I was on a heart monitor. The IV came out a few days later, but the monitor remained. The heart scan showed a slightly enlarged left ventricle.

During my time at St. Luke's I turned thirteen. I became a teenager, but what a way to celebrate my birthday! Still my family, friends, and rehab staff made my situation the best it could be. Counting my stay at Sacred Heart and my rehab at St. Luke's it was twenty-six days. I also spent my first day of 7th grade in rehab. Way too long! I may never know what caused my problems, but I'm back in my ballet pointe shoes and dancing my heart out on my toes!

<hr />

The Story of the Lewan Family

In 2013 I served as the honoree for the Arthritis Foundation's Jingle Bell Run & Walk in Spokane. The JBRW is the foundation's principal fundraising event and is conducted in other cities and towns across the country at the end of each year. My role as the Spokane JBRW Committee spokesman was to help in raising awareness in the community of the impact arthritis has on many Americans, including the 300,000 Katfish, and in asking for donations to the foundation.

At the beginning of my service on the Spokane JBRW Committee, I met Gene Lewan and one of his children, Elyse. Sometime thereafter I learned that she had been diagnosed with JA, but she hadn't spoken to me about it until just before the 2013 JBRW. Both of us were assisting at the event's check-in and packet pickup. During a lull in the process, I struck up a conversation with her. Now a young adult, she has left the ranks of the Katfish—but arthritis has not left her.

Elyse shared with me a little of how it has been to live with JA. It was heartbreaking to listen to her. She then said that her four sisters and one brother suffered from it, too. I was dumbfounded.

Knowing that the Spokane JBRW would need an honoree for the following year, I suggested to the committee that Elyse be asked to serve in this role. Not only did she agree to it, but the entire Lewan family also did. With Gene Lewan's permission here is his story of how the family has been deeply affected by JA.

———

The happiest moments of life are often associated with our children. To see them accomplish goals and go on to lead happy, healthy lives is what every parent wants for their children. I am the father of eight, which includes three sons and five daughters. While the kids were young they were active in many of our community and school events and programs. They had vibrant childhoods.

Ashley is my oldest daughter. She was always a good soccer player. During her freshman year she went out for the high school team. Her knees began to bother her that summer, but her tenacity helped her push on. It soon became apparent that something more was going on, and she had to drop from the team. Doctors couldn't come to a conclusion on the exact cause of her pain and suffering. After several years and multiple doctor visits, Ashley was diagnosed with arthritis and lupus. Later, her two closest sisters, Emily and Elyse, began to exhibit symptoms during their early teens. Elyse was diagnosed with undifferentiated spondyloarthropathy, and Emily was diagnosed with rheumatoid arthritis.

Ashley was placed on medication but couldn't continue the treatments due to complications. Meanwhile her jaw was beginning to show signs of degeneration. Injections of medications into her jaw and other steroid use helped at times but only provided temporary relief. She then switched to a biologic medication for her symptoms. Because of her age, I am no longer able to carry her on my insurance. Ashley's insurance through her job requires such a high co-pay that her treatment has become unaffordable.

In addition to arthritis, Elyse was diagnosed with narcolepsy in high school. She missed many days of school but still finished with a high GPA. She tried to attend college on an academic scholarship, but the combination of her diseases proved too much. She has been declared disabled, but is able to live on her own. She has to fight daily to maintain her disability declaration in order to keep her medicines covered by Medicaid.

Emily, who has RA, postponed college due to migraine headaches. We believe they were the result of the medication she was taking for her arthritis. Since stopping the treatments her migraines have subsided. She works full time and currently takes a biologic medication. Her fingers are beginning to be severely affected, and the joints in her toes are fusing together. Unfortunately, she has few choices due to such severe side effects.

My younger children, Ethan, Mary, and Madilyn were all very young when symptoms started for my oldest daughter, Ashley. Ethan, Mary, and Madi had a different childhood than their older siblings, due to the fact that an extreme amount of time was taken up dealing with different medical visits, trips to specialists, and the cost of all the medications. The fear always lingered that their lives would take the same turn as their sisters'. As fate would have it, they entered their teens and began to show signs of arthritis and autoimmune disease. Mary was diagnosed with RA and other autoimmune disorders and had to have her thyroid removed. She is currently taking biologic medications. Madi was diagnosed with autoimmune arthropathy and her fingers are becoming more severely affected. Ethan has also started showing signs of RA. All three of them work hard and stay active. Mary plays tennis for the high school team, plays oboe in the band, and hopes to pursue marine studies in college. Madi plays flute and is an aspiring artist and writer. Ethan attends college, plays clarinet, and sings and acts in local theater productions. They endure more than they let on to the outside world. At times, though, it's overwhelming.

As a parent it is hard to see your children struggle with this adversity, but I am proud that they are able to dig deep within themselves and carry the load that has been laid upon their shoulders. We have met some very strong and inspirational people who, despite their own chronic illnesses, work hard to help others who are beginning this somber journey. One day I hope that my children and all those affected will be able to live their lives without this physical pain and emotional burden and that they will be able to smile without having to mask the pain.

***

The Story of Isaac Bawden

I met Isaac and his mother, Felicia, through the Spokane JBRW Committee. Isaac is an engaging and determined boy, and he will go far. This is his story as told by Felicia.

***

Isaac is an energetic, happy, charismatic nine year old. From the huge smile on his face, you would not know what battles he has fought in his young life. He was born with E-coli spinal meningitis, which caused hydrocephalus and resulted in a shunt placement. One of the shunts failed, causing a stroke when he was only one year old. This seems more than one person should have to endure in his entire life, but this was far from the end of his battles.

When Isaac was five, we moved to Spokane and started our new life. A couple weeks after the move, Isaac started experiencing excruciating pain in his knee. The pain kept him up at night and we could not find an explanation for it. Several doctors, emergency room visits, x-rays, bone scans, and MRIs couldn't determine the reason this was occurring. Only one month after the pain started Isaac could no longer walk. This was when our visits at Shriners Hospital started. Isaac's leg was casted in an attempt to straighten what we thought were extremely tight muscles in the leg that was affected by the stroke. One month later the cast came off and he was in more pain than ever. With Isaac wheelchair bound, in pain, and still with no answers, we entered a discouraging three months.

Finally, in May of 2012, the doctors at Shriners thought maybe they would cast Isaac again. When they put him under to do the procedure, they could not straighten his leg past 60 degrees. His knee was literally frozen in that position. That is when the possibility of arthritis came into play. With some blood work tests and an evaluation by a rheumatologist, it was determined that there was a very good chance that he had juvenile idiopathic arthritis. So began his lifelong journey with an incurable disease.

Isaac was prescribed methotrexate to treat the arthritis. Slowly, but surely, his swelling reduced and he began to gain mobility. Extensive therapy and continued hard work on his part had him walking the majority of the time by September, just in time for school. He experienced a lot of pain and fatigue during this process, but kept a smile on his face the whole time.

Isaac is one of the most determined kids you will meet. Almost three years after diagnosis, he is just as active as any other nine-year-old boy. He runs cross-country at his school, he plays on a soccer team, and he participates in the school play. He continues taking the methotrexate but has gradually been able to reduce the dosage, which will hopefully help ward off long-term effects.

Since diagnosis, Isaac has become a great advocate for Juvenile Arthritis. He has participated in the Jingle Bell Run/Walk for three years in a row. In March 2014, he went to Washington, D.C., to meet with legislators and make them aware of legislation to help those with arthritis. He continues to be a sparkling, joyful face of arthritis. Don't let his smile fool you though. Arthritis is a difficult disease to live with, and one that he will have to endure his whole life, but if anyone can take on that challenge, it would be Isaac!

The Story of Ashley Smith

Just as I had with the Lewan family and Isaac, I met Ashley through the committee. She is our development coordinator and, I can attest, a go-getter! Now thirty-two, she was diagnosed with RA at eighteen.

My entire adult life I have been trying to figure out this disease and learn how to live with it. A few years ago, I gave up trying to figure arthritis out and decided to focus on living the best life possible while dealing with arthritis.

At age fifteen I was in a car accident. Afterward, I began to experience back pain. I went to the doctor and he couldn't find anything wrong with me, so I went on with life, doing my best to put the pain in the back of my mind. A few months before I turned seventeen I was at a party and an intoxicated man who decided he didn't like my coat picked me up and body slammed me to the ground. My previous back pain then turned into agony, so I went back to the doctor. Again he couldn't find anything wrong. This time, he prescribed physical therapy and said it would help. He was wrong. It didn't help, and sometimes I thought it made the pain worse. I continued to go back to the doctor and he continued to find nothing wrong. They took x-rays and blood tests — you name it, the doctor did it. Finally, one day, he said, "I'm going to do one last blood test and will let you know what I find." A week later a nurse called and asked that I come back in, so I did. Little did I know that my life would be forever changed.

When I went to the appointment, I was sure the doctor would tell me there was nothing wrong. Not this time. He informed me I had tested positive for HLA-B27 and that my RF (rheumatoid factor) was also positive. He then told me that he was referring me to a rheumatologist who could help me. HLA-B27 sounded like a helicopter to me (I still to this day call it the helicopter disease. It is not a disease).

I went to the rheumatology appointment. I don't remember everything from that day, but I do remember the rheumatologist saying, "You have tested positive for HLA-B27 and you have rheumatoid arthritis." After he told me I had arthritis, I remember thinking "Arthritis? What? Isn't that for old people?" Then he pulled out a white sheet of paper and told me my options for medicine. He recommended sulfasalazine and ordered more tests. The main thing I remember from this appointment was when he told me, "This is serious, and if you don't take your medicine you could be in a wheelchair by thirty." I don't know if he said that as a scare tactic because I was young and completely uneducated about arthritis, but I can tell you, I always took my medicine!

Since then, I have been on a handful of medicines including methotrexate and four biologics. I have also married and have two children. I still take my medicine and live my life as normally as possible. My normal regimen just includes medicine that makes me sick from side effects, giving myself shots so I can move my joints, and always feeling tired.

People ask me how arthritis affects my daily life and if I get upset about it. I always tell them, "What people don't ask or understand is how it affects my husband and my kids' lives. Arthritis affects every decision we (my husband and I) make, from our home to how many extracurricular activities our kids can do."

As much as I would like to say I don't allow arthritis to take over my life, I can't. My arthritis was and has been a huge factor since that first rheumatology appointment. Because of the severity of the biological, I couldn't start taking it until after

I was done having kids. When I got to a point that none of the other medications were working and needed the methotrexate and biological, I had to decide I was done having children. When we purchased our last home, we picked a ranch style so I wouldn't have to use the stairs because of morning stiffness. Stairs are not easy in the morning.

When my daughter asks me to do her hair, it takes me a while because my hands and fingers get stiff. Physically I can do anything. If I'm able to move after, that's another story.

I feel like I've learned a lot about life in my thirty-two years, especially that arthritis is a tiring, time-consuming, expensive, and nondiscriminatory disease. I hope someday the younger generations will not have to deal with it.

The Story of Priscilla Hoffman

I met Priscilla because she has an office near mine. She is a sole proprietor, operating as a licensed esthetician and massage therapist. I found out she has psoriatic arthritis, a very painful, chronic, and inflammatory condition that afflicts her entire body. Here is her story.

I am thirty-two years old and learning to live life to the fullest with psoriatic arthritis. It all began when I was young. I had immune-system problems, and was constantly battling tonsillitis, strep throat, and ear infections. I took antibiotics because I didn't know a better way to treat my illnesses, but the antibiotics were ruining my immune system. Then at age fifteen my joints started to flare up. I would wake up with a knee or shoulder so swollen that I suffered a lot of pain.

I saw many different doctors who diagnosed tendonitis, bursitis, and even a torn ACL, but I had never had any injuries to cause my pain and inflammation. They prescribed physical therapy, pain medications, and anti-inflammatories, but none of them helped. I still kept going to the doctor, but I was beside myself, frustrated and confused. I was then denied care because I was labeled a "drug seeker." One rheumatologist even told me there was nothing wrong because my rheumatoid factor was negative. Finally, my chiropractor knew it was something deeper that she couldn't treat. After learning my history of childhood illnesses of psoriasis and eczema, she referred me to another rheumatologist. At last, at age twenty-five, I had a diagnosis: psoriatic arthritis — but I was devastated!

At the same time, however, it was nice to hear that I was not crazy any more. I was terrified, though, when I learned more about psoriatic arthritis. I was told I would probably be crippled in the next ten years if I did not act fast so my rheumatologist started me on biological drugs. I took sulfasalazine and Enbrel. There wasn't much improvement and my flare-ups kept me from my practice. I also tried Remicade, another biological, and spent thousands of dollars for co-pays and deductibles. Nothing! I went back to Enbrel, steroids, and cortisone injections. My work got more unbearable and I ended up needing my hand surgically reconstructed to be able to continue working.

Still, I just kept getting sick. I knew the risks of being on all of these drugs, but I didn't care. I would try anything to not be in the kind of pain I was suffering. That was until the drugs almost killed me. My immune system was so shot from the immunosuppressant therapy that I wasn't able to heal from the simplest infections, such as an ingrown toenail and a septic tooth abscess. Oral antibiotics didn't kick in and I just got sicker. After a week of going to the doctor for injections to keep me out of the hospital, I finally started to recover. That was my wake-up call.

I still ended up in the ER and felt like dying. The doctor said, "Well, as soon as you recover from this, get back on Enbrel."

I said, "Are you kidding me? Those drugs are killing me!" That was when I broke down and sought God. I asked Him to show me how to care for this body He's given me and how to restore it to how He originally created it to be.

After a lot of research I realized how messed up my gut was from all of the antibiotics. The immune system originates from the gut. No more covering up symptoms for me! I wanted to go straight to the cause of my arthritis and cure it. I tried everything my doctors recommended and it was time for a real change. I researched how to restore my gut through diet change, paleo/anti-inflammatory nutrition, yoga, and supplements of probiotics, quality vitamins, and natural anti-inflammatories. I then started to see real change. After three months of dedication to caring for myself I actually felt like a normal human being without arthritis!

I still have occasional flare-ups, especially when I get off track and don't care for my body like God showed me to do, but I no longer feel defined by my disease. That's not who I am or who God has called me to be. I no longer lay in bed for days at a time feeling depressed that I will be crippled or die. God has given me the strength to press on even through flare-ups. I will not give up on life. I am called to a much bigger purpose of serving and loving people, and I can't fulfill that purpose if I choose to stay in bed wallowing in my suffering and loaded up on drugs. I don't believe that is the purpose for anyone's life. Don't give up on your fight!

The Story of Annie Jones

I met Annie through Ashley Smith. Both had learned of each other through social media. Annie is a yoga instructor and works with a variety of clientele, including young children ranging from two-year-olds to five-year-olds, but what is most interesting is her story about living with RA and overcoming it to help others through yoga. Here is her story as told by her husband Michael.

Tenaciousness has never been my strong suit. I've been described as many things in my lifetime, mostly with adjectives synonymous with different types of rodents, reptiles, and raunchy plastic gag gifts. I have, however, always admired this insistent quality from afar. That is, I had admired tenaciousness from afar — until I met Annie. Since meeting Annie, I've come to a whole new appreciation for this amazing quality. Not only does she fit the description, she redefines it.

Annie was diagnosed with rheumatoid arthritis seven years ago... she turns thirty this year. I can only speak from my perspective on the matter — with my limited knowledge of this inflammatory disorder I'm hardly an expert — but she was too damn young to be diagnosed with this disease. Seven years into it, I've seen Annie master many things in her life. She's conquered just about every curveball thrown her way because of her RA and seems to get stronger and more pertinacious with every obstacle put in front of her. I fell in love with this woman years ago, before I knew she would become the person she is today. I would never claim to be grateful for RA being introduced into my life through the person I love most, but I will say that having the opportunity to watch that person battle so hard with something so extremely daunting has turned me into someone I could have only hoped to be growing up as a wild, carefree, and completely ignorant little plastic gag gift.

When I met Annie, I admit she intimidated me. This girl was something special and unquestionably out of my league: gorgeous, intelligent, kind, friendly, with an obvious sense of self-confidence and strength. Most important, she was willing to give me the time of day. Don't get me wrong: I wasn't under any impression that I would land a date with this girl, let alone hold a conversation with her stimulating enough to spark some interest on her part. It was satisfying enough knowing I'd get to go to work every day and receive any kind of attention from someone so clearly in control of everything that I looked for in a human being.

I was working as a sous-chef in a corporate food trough, and Annie was serving tables at the same restaurant. In my mind, at the very least I had a chef coat with my name on it, so I wouldn't have to deal with the inevitable awkward moment that I would be swimming in her beautiful brown eyes when I realized that she couldn't quite put a name to my face. Luckily, that moment never happened. Instead, I fought every reasonable voice in my head and asked this vision of perfection out on a date, and in the same moment of delusion, she fought every reasonable voice in her head and agreed to that date.

After months of begging and blackmailing, I finally convinced Annie to admit to herself that we were dating. In my mind, I had accomplished life's ultimate goal: I had mastered the art of hypnosis and convinced this woman with movie star looks — and personality to spare — to actually enjoy being around me. We were young and in love… we, not just I! Every crazy idea I threw at her she doubled down on. Every stupid adventure I took her on she somehow transformed into an amazing, life-changing experience. The gravy train had departed the station and we were on it with a never-ending supply of biscuits.

The morning Annie woke up and couldn't get out of bed wasn't especially traumatizing or scary. In fact, I was happy to have a day to pamper her and nurse her back to perfect health, and then to bask in the glory that was I. The day of discomfort turned into a week of excruciating pain, and the week turned into a month. She was making every attempt to be as tough as she possibly could, but there was no hiding it.

Every morning Annie would wake up as if she had invisible weights strapped to her body. After mustering the strength to even make an attempt to get out of bed, she would start to wiggle toward the edge of the mattress. Once she had accomplished what seemed to be an impossible task of wiggling twelve inches to the left, she would slide out of bed and fall to the floor as if she were avoiding a high-tech infrared security system that you might see in a bank-heist movie. At this point she needed help to do anything else. Don't get the wrong impression, because this girl has a pain threshold that would rival a prizefighter's. This wasn't weakness. This was a human being putting up her best fight just to get out of bed in the morning. The torture of getting dressed was simply too much.

In a perfect world we could all stroll around naked; in a perfect world no one would have to wake up in the morning paralyzed with pain. At the time, we lived in Scottsdale, Arizona, and had the benefit of wearing very little clothing and having a pool within crawling distance. It didn't quite provide comfort, but it at least took away the struggle of having to fight gravity.

Annie had become a shell of her former self. Her tall, slender frame was hunched over. Her perfectly sculpted arms were curled in toward her body, and she walked as if she were on an endless trail of glass shards. This strong, independent woman couldn't open a can or bottle, let alone turn a doorknob or open a car door on her own. We hadn't quite been dating for a year, but I knew how much it took for Annie to swallow her pride and ask for help in everything that she was doing.

For months Annie dealt with this pain. For months, every day was a struggle to get up, to get moving, and to battle a day full of agonizing pain. We were completely in the dark, with no idea of what this debilitating disease was or how it seemingly appeared out of nowhere. She didn't have health insurance, and the fear of the endless possibilities of what was slowly beating her down was terrifying for both of us. The only thing worse than watching her struggle through every day, both physically and mentally, was the fact that there was absolutely nothing I could do to help relieve any of that pain. The illness began to consume us.

In hindsight I'm ashamed of myself for allowing frustration to show. I'm embarrassed that during this time that the love of my life was suffering the most, I couldn't be stronger. Instead, I began to feel sorry for myself. In my most selfish moments, Annie could read the frustration on my face, which led to more confusion and pain. I was struggling with my helplessness. There had to be more that I could do than simply open cans, bottles, and doors for her — but what?

I've had a lifelong habit of making bad things worse, and here, when Annie needed me the most, I was in my finest hour of destruction. Instead of throwing in the towel on me, as I was beginning to do with Annie, she decided to fight — to fight me and to fight this disease that I was allowing to plague our relationship. It was hands down the best decision I never made.

Annie began the fight against her arthritis with her plastic turd of a boyfriend. Instead of allowing my silent frustration, she demanded communication. Instead of trying to hide her pain, both physically and emotionally, she put it all out on the table. We fought, we cried, and we made up our minds to fight this thing together. There was no hiding from this, only conquering it. I can only imagine a world where I possess the courage that it took her to take control of every aspect of her life, but she did it without a flinch. We began to look into every possibility of what this illness could be. We reached out to family and friends for any help that they might be able to offer. The seed had been sown and the tenacity was growing.

We soon moved from Arizona, where we met, to New Mexico. I had grown up in New Mexico and had accepted a job offer in Albuquerque where my family was living. This move would end up being a major catalyst in our journey together. Annie began to look at options for any kind of assistance we might be eligible for in New Mexico. She found her answer through the University Hospital in Albuquerque. Within a month of being there, she received a diagnosis: rheumatoid arthritis. With the terrible discovery of a lifelong disease came the short-term relief of finding some sort of solution for the physical pain. Unfortunately, a solution wasn't a cure, nor was it anything close to permanent.

The road to answers began with a cocktail of drugs. I couldn't possibly recall, spell, or correctly pronounce the assortment of drugs that Annie was put on, but I'll try. It began with

Prednisone, and moved to Plaquenil and then Methotrexate. Along with the nausea, which went hand-in-hand with these drugs, was the discovery that they weren't meant for someone Annie's age. With plans to start a family and lead as healthy a life as possible, it was time to start looking for other options.

Annie's specialist started her on Enbrel, which we were extremely hopeful about. It certainly seemed like the best option. Unquestionably, the drugs were helping with her pain, along with the knowledge of having some idea of what we were up against. It was finally time to focus our attention on something, anything, that wasn't RA related.

Our hopes of starting a family together would soon come to fruition. Along with the excitement of having a baby on the way was the sense of optimism that Annie might get some relief from her RA during pregnancy. From what we had researched and heard through experts on the subject, the symptoms of RA would likely recede during her pregnancy. Unfortunately, once again luck would not be on her side. Not only did she still experience the same debilitating pain that she had grown accustomed to, but she also would have to avoid any of the drugs that might be helping her with the pain.

Like the champ she is, Annie would fight her way through the pregnancy with almost no complaints. I remember the night she went into labor. One of her main priorities was making sure she had Enbrel the moment she gave birth. It wasn't the fear of giving birth that she was focused on, but the relief of pain from her arthritis that was consuming her thoughts. We would have a baby boy, Miles, and be married in the same year. Within two years of moving to New Mexico, it looked like we were boarding the gravy train again.

Annie's RA was never out of sight or out of mind. After giving birth to Miles, it seemed as if she was out of the frying pan and into the fire. Her pain would return and the drugs didn't seem to be working as well as they had in the past. The feelings of frustration were back. She was on her fourth year of battling this illness and it would seem like a lifetime. So what did she do? She fought harder. She found levels of tenacity that I never knew existed. If drugs weren't the answer, a complete change of lifestyle was in order.

This is the part of the story that I introduce a new character. This is the second coming of Annie Jones. If you thought the first Annie was amazing, wait until you meet the new version. It began with a complete overhaul of her diet. She eliminated basically everything out of her daily intake, save a limited amount of fruits, vegetables, and chicken. After months of this, she began to slowly introduce one item of food at a time, paying close attention to how her body would respond to it. Eventually she would settle on completely eliminating nightshades (look it up if you aren't already familiar with it) because of their glycoalkaloids, and gluten. She avoids refined sugar, for the most part, as well as citrus, dairy, and most red meats. She began to truly understand her body and how it responded to everything she put in it. Anything she consumed that she felt resulted in a flare up of her RA was immediately removed from her life. It seemed to be working. She was feeling better, looking better, and gaining confidence.

The next step in Annie's battle with RA would arguably be the most important... and I'm not sure that it's really arguable. She began to practice yoga. It started as an experiment of sorts; another level of understanding her body and pushing it to its limit. What it turned into was something else entirely. She began to practice daily, then several times a day. Eventually, she decided to put in the hours and become a yoga instructor.

Becoming a yoga instructor wasn't simply an aspiration that Annie had to perfect her practice or to deepen her understanding of the art. Her true intention is to spread the love. In yoga she found something that truly helped heal her, both physically and mentally. She is the healthiest and strongest that she has ever been. By no means has her pain from RA magically disappeared. Nor has the fear of what the future might hold for her, but through her personal strength and her newfound love of yoga, she has come to accept the hand that she's been dealt in life. Yoga has become the most central part of what Annie attributes to her success in overcoming RA (besides her stud of a husband, of course).

When I met Annie, I knew I had found the perfect specimen of a woman. She is everything a man could ask for. Every ounce of this beautiful woman is physically desirable, and if you can manage to keep up with her intellectually, then you've earned the right to fall in love. The trick is to fall in love twice. When you realize the strength it takes to fight rheumatoid arthritis, and the defiance it takes to not let it rule your life, you have no choice but to love the hero in the heat of the battle.

I've given Annie many titles since I've met her (plastic turd never made the list), but "tenacious" is the title she's earned at every turn. Tenacity is the quality that every relationship needs to survive. Tenacity is the conqueror of all things. Because of tenacity, rheumatoid arthritis cannot possibly win.

Christina, Isaac, the Lewan family, Ashley, Priscilla, and Annie are indeed profiles in courage. Their indomitable spirit has enabled them to face the vicissitudes of arthritis with self-possession, confidence, and resolution. They have been severely challenged by their condition, and yet they have not given into it. True grit indeed! Their stories and those of other Katfish inspire me to continue on the journey to the cure.

Chapter 25

The Teaching of Frida Kahlo

I hope the exit is joyful and I hope never to come back.
—Frida Kahlo

When the great Mexican artist Frida Kahlo wrote these desperate yet hopeful words on July 9, 1954, I turned seven years of age. Four days later Frida died. Her life is a study of pain and passion. Her paintings are almost exclusively devoted to how the tragedies she suffered her entire adult life consumed her. She was horribly injured in a bus accident at the age of eighteen. During the course of her life, she endured more than thirty-five operations. The self-portraits of her suffering hit me so hard that on reflection I know exactly what she went through emotionally. She is a kindred spirit. I identify with Frida.

I learned about Frida through a film of her life. Salma Hayek portrayed this amazing woman. I was captivated. For further details, I urge the reader to view the classic, *Frida*. During the course of my yoga instruction by Natalie Gauvin, who is also an artist, I said I knew how Frida felt. I also said to Natalie that Frida's final diary entry was something I thought about very much. Yoga was the last resort and I believed that if it didn't work, I hoped my end was near. I have lived a long life for a Katfish, and I should have died by now.

After listening to me about Frida's last words and how I dwelt on them, Natalie advised me to consider that Frida's life, painful as it was, is an inspiration. Her pain produced such moving self-portraits that the flipside of her nature was her passion. She was Janus. To me this Roman god signifies that good times and bad times are part of life, so deal with them until it's over.

With yoga I have at last turned the corner. Because of it I am so much better physically, mentally, and spiritually. I now believe I will live a long time. This is good. I can concentrate on raising awareness about juvenile arthritis and finding the cure for it. My pain is essential for my passion and my passion is essential for my memoir. Both help me inspire Katfish to carry on the best way they can.

Chapter 26

Earnestly Do I Hope

Whatever happened to polio?
—Smithsonian Institute

I first encountered this question at an exhibition in the National Museum of American History. Funded by the March of Dimes, the principal sponsor, and by Rotary International and the Salk Institute for Biological Studies, this fiftieth-year commemorative event was about the announcement of Dr. Jonas Salk's polio vaccine in 1955, what came before it, and the lasting changes that polio, and the people who had it, created in American culture.

As I walked through the exhibition, I was reminded of my own childhood vaccinations against the most notorious disease of the 20th century before AIDS confronted this country. First reported in the United States in 1894, polio, also known as infantile paralysis, occurred in the summer and plagued communities, regardless of geographic region, economic status, or population density. No one understood how or why people got it. Children were the most frequently affected and, if they survived, could face a life with paralyzed limbs and other permanent disabilities. No device is more associated with the disease than the "iron lung." For a person whose breathing muscles had been paralyzed by the virus, this machine maintained respiration artificially until the patient could breathe independently.

Hailed as a medical miracle, the development of the Salk vaccine would not have been possible without the heroic "Polio Pioneers," children in the first three grades of elementary school selected to test the effectiveness of the vaccine. Although I was eligible to be a Polio Pioneer in 1954, my school was not chosen as one of the 215 test sites. Nevertheless, clinical trials funded by the March of Dimes targeted 1.8 million children. By receiving a series of injections, these "little guinea pigs" paved the way for approval of Salk's discovery and led to the eradication of polio, both at home and abroad.

In 2009, I was honored with the Arthritis Foundation's Inspirational Leadership award for the Pacific Northwest Chapter. In my acceptance remarks, I credited President Franklin Roosevelt as one of the individuals who inspired me to carry on as an advocate for the cure of arthritis. It was his personal battle with polio that focused the nation's attention on effectively dealing with this disease, but it also took the time, energy, and resources of individuals, organizations, and the government to defeat it. At the conclusion, I said:

"Earnestly do I hope we can mirror the success story about polio and pose a similar question in our own commemorative victory: 'Whatever happened to arthritis?'"

Chapter 27

The Great Task Remaining Before Us: The Cure

People are waiting for cues from you. Lead them well!
—Chinese fortune cookie

It is to Katfish I look for the answer to "Whatever happened to juvenile arthritis?" You are the pathfinders who will finish the great task remaining before us and lead us well to the cure for juvenile arthritis. You are like the Polio Pioneers. Without the valuable contributions of these young heroes, eradicating polio would have been much harder to accomplish; but your goal must not be mass vaccination. When you reach the end of your journey, the cure for juvenile arthritis must be safe, effective, and affordable.

The proof for such a proposition is promising. A cure for hepatitis C has been at long last developed. Twenty-five years after scientists first discovered this virus, doctors are declaring victory over an infection that afflicts more than 3 million Americans and kills more of them than AIDS.

The stories of Kelly Norris, Taylor Bruce, Riley Gonzales, Christina McCarty, Isaac Bawden, Ashley Smith, the Lewan family, Priscilla Hoffman, and Annie Jones, as well as my own, are proof that expensive pharmaceutical drugs developed for inflammatory arthritis in adults, not Katfish, are filled with risks Katfish should never have to think about, let alone deal with, especially when you cannot provide "informed consent" for yourselves; instead, your dear parents must make this very hard decision.

With just 250 pediatric rheumatologists to treat 300,000 Katfish, time is of the utmost essence to find the cure for juvenile arthritis. Underscoring the urgency to act now is that present treatments only control juvenile arthritis. Even if it's put into remission with drugs developed for adults, the condition is dormant, not extinct. Add to this the risks, both known and unknown, of the powerful yet potentially dangerous juvenile arthritis treatments and the extremely burdensome expense of biological medications, and Katfish must champion their own cause to find a safe, effective, and affordable cure.

The most important reason for finishing The Great Task Remaining Before Us now is the avoidance of a life filled with the pain, suffering, and mental anguish juvenile arthritis inflicts on the mind, body, and spirit. Therefore, Katfish, in the words of President John Quincy Adams: "If your actions inspire others to dream more, learn more, do more, and become more, you are a leader."

Be a juvenile arthritis pathfinder and lead us well on the Journey to the Cure!

Epilogue

When I started on my path of living with arthritis, I had no cues about what to do. As a child of eleven in 1959, I could not comprehend that the rest of my life had changed forever. All I wanted then, and for many years thereafter, was a return to normalcy—a healthy body not limited by chronic pain, suffering, and disability, but such was not to be. It would take a long time for me to accept this harsh reality and deal with it properly. Now, in my sixty-eighth year, I believe I have.

Fifty-seven years of living with arthritis have taken their toll. The disease, the adverse health conditions caused by it, and some of the treatments I've tried have left me with permanent disability and deformity. The prospect of further surgery looms larger as a result, and the pain nags me daily. Given this lengthy legacy of arthritis and that more of my path lies behind than ahead, I sometimes call to mind the cogent warning the poet Virgil gave many centuries ago when he said, "Death plucks my ear and says, 'Live—I am coming!'"

On his 90th birthday, Oliver Wendell Holmes, an associate justice of the U.S. Supreme Court, cited Virgil's admonition during a celebration of this special occasion. Before his 30-year tenure on the country's high court bench began, Holmes had been a soldier, lawyer, professor, and state court judge. A prodigious person by nature, Holmes understood that one's work is never done while the power to work remains. "For to live is to function. That is all there is in living."

Please heed the advice of Jagger and Richards. I know I have, and I am far richer in my mind, body, and spirit because of the blessing of arthritis, for I am the sum of my life experiences and my relationships—past, present, and to come. In addition to my family and friends, I appreciate the following individuals who also helped me on my path:

My manuscript readers, Shirley and Bob Pederson, Robert Schlim, S.J., Maureen McGuire, Ashley Lewan, Merri Hartse, Jon Stevenson, M.D., Helen Emery, M.D., Jeanne McCarty, Scott Weaver, Johanna Lindsay, Wendy P. Cossette, and Rep. Cathy McMorris Rodgers;

My secretary, Debra Clary;

My colleagues, Bill Maxey, Keith Briggs, Ken Isserlis, Larry Weiser, Bob Morozzo, and Byron Walters;

My long-distance swimming support team, Benita and Bob Galland; and

My literary agent, Steve Bruno.

Thus, while I still have "all my marbles," coupled with the ability to function physically and aided by my family and friends, I shall blaze on my path to raise awareness about juvenile arthritis. As I said at the beginning of my tale, I hope to continue helping on the Journey to the Cure for Juvenile Arthritis, thereby making the Katfish like the dinosaur—a thing of the past!

Author's Note

Inspiration for writing my memoir came from many sources, one of them Professor William Prosser. In the preface to his delightful and informative primer, *The Law of Torts*, Professor Prosser expressed his gratitude, together with his apologies, to able and distinguished writers whose ideas he unblushingly appropriated in penning his classic hornbook. He then concluded: "A packrat is at best a collector, and no heroic figure; and the most that can be said for him is that he sometimes chooses well."

Like Prosser's packrat, I hope I have sometimes chosen well from the inspirational stories of the Katfish, as well as from my own personal experiences, to write this one pathfinder's way of living with arthritis.

Now I lay down my pen and, for just a little while, cease upon my labor of love.

The Rheumatoid Arthritis Project Summary

The Rheumatoid Arthritis Project, a nonprofit 501©(3) Washington corporation was formed in 2004. Its mission is to raise awareness about juvenile arthritis and to help in finding the cure. A board of trustees manages the affairs of the project, which consist of helping Katfish in the Inland Northwest community. Such assistance encompasses safe, effective, and affordable treatments, including non-medical, non-surgical modalities of hydrotherapy, ai chi, swimming, and other noninvasive complementary healthcare practices. Profits from the sale of *Tale of an Old Katfish* will be used by the board to implement the project's mission.

Resources

Angell, Marcia, M.D. *The Truth About the Drug Companies: How They Deceive Us and What to Do About It.* Random House, 2004.

Arthritis Foundation, www.arthritis.org

Arthritis Foundation's Guide to Good Living With Rheumatoid Arthritis, 1999.

Arthritis Foundation's Arthritis Friendly Yoga. DVD, 2014.

Childhood Arthritis and Rheumatology Research Alliance (CARRA), www.carragroup.org

Goozner, Merrill. *The $800 Million Pill: The Truth behind the Cost of New Drugs.* The University of California Press, 2004.

Horstman, Judith. Arthritis Foundation's Guide to Alternative Therapies, 1999.

Huff, Charlotte. *Raising a Child With Arthritis, A Parent's Guide.* Arthritis Foundation, 2012.

Kids Get Arthritis Too, www.kidsgetarthritistoo.org

National Center for Complementary and Alternative Medicine, www.nccam.nih.gov

National Institute for Arthritis, Musculoskeletal, and Skin Diseases, www.niams.nih.gov

"Rheumatoid Arthritis and Complementary and Alternative Medicine," www.nccam.nih.gov

About the Author

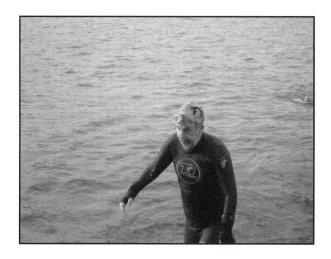

John P. Lynch has had rheumatoid arthritis since 1959. He and his wife, Vivian, have two children, Monica and Matt, and three grandchildren, Corinne, Lauren, and Ryan. Monica is a pharmacist and Matt is a quality assurance manager.

John holds a bachelor's degree in chemistry from the University of Washington, an MBA from the University of Oregon, and a juris doctor from Gonzaga University. In addition to being an emeritus member of the Washington State Bar Association, he has a CPA certificate from the Washington State Board of Accountancy.

From 1978 to 2007 John was in the private practice of law as a sole proprietor, specializing in plaintiff personal injury cases, estate planning, and probate. In 2004, he formed The Rheumatoid Arthritis Project, a nonprofit organization whose mission is to help find the cure for juvenile arthritis.

Since 2001 John has been a volunteer advocate for the Great West Region of the Arthritis Foundation. The region has honored him with its 2002 Advocacy Award and 2009 Inspirational Leadership Award. In 2013 he was the region's honoree for the Spokane Jingle Bell Run & Walk. Through the foundation's annual advocacy summits in Washington, D.C., John and other advocates helped secure Medicare coverage of self-injected biological drugs for inflammatory arthritis. In the U.S. Congress and state legislatures, they raise awareness about arthritis, especially juvenile arthritis, advocating for the appropriation of sufficient public resources to prevent, control, and cure this chronic, painful, and disabling condition.